HEAD TO TOE HEALING

The Discovery That Led To The Most Healing Results Ever Recorded on Video

The 14th Published Book By

Dr. Kevin Reese, PhD, PAS, INHC, DS

Copyright © 2025

www.DRKEVINREESE.com

Head To Toe Healing

Seven Thirty Enterprises LLC

ISBN: 979-8-9896423-1-1

Copyright © 2025

All rights reserved. This book or any portion thereof may not be reproduced unless the author is given credit.

No information in this book is intended as a substitute for the medical advice of a licensed physician. Kevin Reese, PhD, PAS, INHC, DS is NOT a licensed physician. Kevin Reese is a doctor of philosophy (phd) and is known as a head to toe healer who educates others on the topic of health and wellness.

Dr. Reese does not diagnose, treat or cure diseases, instead he gives assessments, provides education and gives recommendations based on the belief that the human body is divinely designed to heal itself.

You should check with your licensed primary care physician anytime you change diet or exercise. You should also seek medical care if you have an infection, a new injury or are in urgent need of attention.

Although the author and publisher have made every effort to ensure that the information in this book was correct at press time, the author and publisher do not assume and hereby disclaim any liability to any party for any loss, damage, or disruptions caused by errors or omissions, whether such errors or omissions result from negligence or any other cause.

The writings in this book are meant for educational purposes. If you take any advice from this book, you do so at your own discretion.

Table of Contents

Table Of Contents ---- *3*

The Discovery ---- *6*

14-Hour Long Gallbladder Pain Completely Gone ---- *17*

Bulging Discs Gone, Frozen Shoulder Gone & Immobility Gone ---- *21*

Asthma Gone, Allergies Gone And Eczema Gone ---- *24*

Costochondritis Gone, Plantar Fasciitis Gone, Numbness In Legs Gone, Cracked Heels Gone, Age Spots Disappearing ---- *26*

Insomnia Gone ---- *28*

Hip Pain Gone In 2 Weeks ---- *30*

Psoriasis Gone In 30 Days ---- *32*

Pcos, Diabetes, Gut Issues, Body Pain & Duck Feet Gone ---- *34*

Frozen Shoulder Gone & Depression Gone ---- *39*

Gray Hair And Age Spots Gone? ---- *41*

Hot Flashes Eliminated, Feet Pain Gone, Back Pain Gone, And Sleep Restored ---- *43*

Sciatica Pain Gone In 70 Days ---- *45*

Tinnitus Gone, Vertigo Gone, Jaw Clicking Gone, Ibs Gone And Ear Unblocked ---- *48*

Acid Reflux Gone, Knee Pain Gone, Migraines Gone, Baldness Gone, Brain Fog Gone, And Grew Half Of An Inch!? ---- *50*

Hashimoto's Symptoms Reduced And Knee Pain Gone ---- *53*

Fibroids Gone, Psoriasis Gone And Migraines Gone ---- *55*

Off Blood Pressure Meds And Hormone Replacement Therapy (Hrt) ---- *57*

No More Walking Cane! ---- *59*

Numbness Gone, Raynaud's Gone, Irregular Heartbeat Gone In 60 Days. No More Neck Brace Or Er Visits ---- *61*

Kidney Function Restored. Chronic Constipation, Astigmatism, And Nodules Gone. All Blood Tests Improved Drastically. ------ 63

Arthritic Hip Pain Gone In 30 Days, Gerd Gone, Neuropathy Pain Disappearing ------ 76

Diabetes Gone ------ 79

40 Symptoms Down To Just 10 Symptoms ------ 81

Knee Clicking Gone, Walking Pattern Restored ------ 83

Age Spots Gone, Panic Attacks Gone, Frozen Shoulder Gone, Migraines Gone, Low Blood Sugar Gone ------ 85

All Digestive Symptoms Massively Improving ------ 87

No Walker Needed, Sciatica Is Gone ------ 89

Hernia Hump Gone ------ 91

Period Pain Gone, Migraines Gone, Acne Gone, Constipation Gone ------ 93

Tmj Gone, Migraines Gone And Back Pain Gone ------ 95

Ulcerative Colitis Gone! ------ 101

Vocal Cord Regenerated ------ 103

Blood Sugar Down 154 Points ------ 106

Allergies Gone & Kidney Pain Gone ------ 108

Hand Pain Gone And Brain Fog Gone In 50 Days ------ 110

Chronic Stomach Pain Gone And Skin Blemishes Gone ------ 112

Pregnant Women Given 3 Months To Live... ------ 114

Scoliosis Reversing In 70-Year-Old Woman! ------ 133

Plantar Fasciitis Gone And Knee Pain Gone ------ 135

Hypertension, Cysts, Stomach Pain, Migraines Gone ------ 138

Conquering Depression, Arthritis, And Weight Loss: Dr. Reese's 120-Day Challenge Transformed My Life ------ 140

Arthritis Gone In 30 Days ------ 142

Vertigo Gone, Heart Palpitations Gone, Heart Pain Gone, Digestive Issues Gone ------ 149

Man Credits Dr. Reese For Life-Changing Recovery From Brain Tumor -- 151

Sciatica Gone In 60 Days, Gums Regenerating, Can Tie Shoes Again ----- 155

Low Back Pain Gone --- 158

Debilitating Migraines Gone And Sinus Infections Gone -------------------- 160

Down 30 Lbs From Just The Poor 4 Foods! --------------------------------- 162

Insomnia Gone -- 164

Hip Pain Gone And Lower Back Pain Gone--------------------------------- 166

Neuropathy Gone In 4 Days!? --- 168

Off Thyroid Meds And Lost 30lbs -- 170

No Pain Anywhere And Cholesterol Lowered ------------------------------ 173

Ibs Gone, Pancreatitis Gone, Ulcers Gone----------------------------------- 175

Fatty Liver Gone, High Blood Pressure Gone, High Cholesterol Gone ----- 177

Sciatica Gone -- 179

Chronic Kidney Dysfunction Gone, Stomach Cramping Gone, High Triglycerides Gone --- 181

Running Again...Down 20+ Pounds And Sleeping Great!--------------------- 183

Sciatica Gone, Acid Reflux Gone, Inflammation Gone, Weight Reduced 185

Debilitating Migraines Gone, Off 16 Meds ---------------------------------- 187

Head To Toe Healing --- 212

Q & A With Dr. Reese-- 216

About The Author -- 229

The Discovery

Head To Toe Healing was an evolution that happened over the course of nearly 15 years. It all started in 2010 when I became a detoxification health practitioner who helped people overcome chronic conditions.

Some of my biggest testimonials happened back then, including Kim, who was told she was going to die at childbirth because of a tumor blocking the birth canal. Her son is now in middle school. Or Grissel who had such bad migraines that she couldn't leave her house. She is happily migraine free a decade later.

However, with the detox business comes the pressure of dealing with the "healing crisis." This is a term used when the body releases toxins too quickly and the body reacts. I had to deal with constant body rashes, flu-like symptoms, horrible headaches, globs of goo fallign out of vagina's (it was known to happen) and more.

Not to mention parasites. Yep. You haven't lived until you see a worm come out of your booty. Whipworms, fluke worms, tape worms and more.

Of course the hot trend was the practice of fasting. I myself experimented heavily. I remember doing 7 days on nothing but water and tea. The feeling I had was horrible. It's like I had the flu. I realized that water was too much, so I did 10 days on juice. This went better. Then I did 30 days on nothing but fruits and veggies. Ok, pretty good. Then I did 30 days of just juice. I even did 10 days of grapes and 30 days of melons. Eventually I progressed to living on nothing but juice every winter. 100 days at a time. Yes, it was cold.

This was my life. Everything was detox and cleansing.

I noticed that my clients did get better but it wasn't sustainable. Everyone crashed and burned inside of 6 months. I also noticed that I crashed and burned. It was a cycle. Fast, feel good, then binge food, then fast again. Was this an eating disorder?

Later in my career as a health practitioner, I noticed a new trend. It was a bunch of my colleagues leaving the detox movement and eating animal products. I knew these were not dumb people so there must have been something to it. I investigated.

While I investigated, tragedy struck. A colleague of mine died. She was one of the more known detoxification practitioners but apparently and allegedly she took it too far.

Then a very known raw vegan personality announced something unthinkable. He got sick and had to have his colon removed. What!? How!?

It was becoming obvious this detoxification thing was not right.

In 2018, I shut down my practice.

I was burnt out, but not just from the harsh reality of detox but also by the fact that I wasn't making good money. It was a struggle. I didn't have a huge audience on social media and the money I was making, like detox, was not sustainable.

My whole identity was on the line. Who was I as a health practitioner?

Here's the part that was interesting. I was attending a distant learning school earning a doctorate in nutrition. I'm sure this also contributed to my burn out because it was so tedious. By the time my degree was delivered to me (yes through the mail) I quit being a health practitioner. So now I'm looking at this degree, which was basically a receipt, and wondering what the point was.

My plan was to work on my Sunlight Sonny children's book. It was a safe and noble project because all it taught was getting children off of junk food. I could make a change with this!

I wanted to expand it into a whole universe, like Star Wars or Marvel Comics. However, the issue was the money. I needed funds to get this off the ground and I didn't have it. I also didn't have a big enough following on social media to raise funds. I was in a pickle.

It wasn't long before something called me back to the health game. While I was having some down time, I started studying the 90 essential nutrients from Dr. Joel Wallach. His work was fascinating because it started with him being a world class veterinarian. He would help animals heal through nutrition and he eventually started helping humans in the same way.

Wallach had a list of the "bad foods" not to eat. I simplified them into 4 foods which became known as the "poor 4 foods." Then I had a realization. The people I was helping with detoxification through those 8 years weren't getting better because of the detox, it was because they were not eating the "poor 4 foods." Next epiphany: the reason detox wasn't sustainable was because eventually the body needed to be replenished with those 90 essential nutrients.

Ahh. So, it's a tag-team effort. Get off the "poor 4 foods" and get on the 90 essential nutrients. They go together! Got it.

During this time, my body started physically breaking down. My back, my shoulders, my hands. This was from decades of being at the computer slumped over. I tried chiropractors, osteopaths and massages and nothing helped. The creams and oils also failed. Eventually I cracked and went to my primary care physician and he sent me to physical therapy.

Physical therapy helped a little but it more so gave me an idea. I remember laying on the table being stretched out and realizing that nutrition can't fix everything. There's a missing piece to health. It's the musculoskeletal system.

I started researching and found Pete Eogscue who was a Marine who was injured in battle. After being shot in war, he, like me, went on a hunt to fix his musculoskeletal issues. He ended up reading the massive book, Grey's Anatomy and realizing the body is a whole unit, it's connected. He simplified the musculoskeletal system and created a new method called postural therapy. It made complete sense, to get the muscles back in order because the muscles move the bones. You see, when the bones get out of alignment, you walk around earth or sit at your computer and the muscles lock you in that position. This position is called posture.

After years of discomfort, I was relieved in just 3 weeks of doing postural therapy daily. I was so impressed that I had to learn this method. So guess what I did at 40 something years old. I went back to school!

It was so hard. The musculoskeletal system is very complicated because there are 600 or so muscles and 200 or so bones. Then let's add in tendons, ligaments and fascia tissue. This school made me want to bash my head against a wall, but I did it.

As I was in school I would meet people who healed themselves just from postural therapy. One guy I met was in a wheelchair and got himself walking and running again. This amazed me because he didn't change his diet at all. In fact, he was obese! It was 100% postural therapy that helped him. I knew that I had truly stumbled on the missing link.

Soon, I was trained to deal with musculoskeletal issues like herniated discs, bunions, frozen shoulder, tennis elbow, cartilage loss and more. My knowledge expanded in a major way.

Soon, I met a guy who sent me down another path. We were talking about pain and he told me that his horrible back pain wasn't relieved until he addressed some emotional issues. Ah. Another healing, but without nutrition or postural therapy. I went home and studied some more. This is when I came across Dr. John Sarno. He was an MD who went rogue and started teaching people to address their mind in order to heal their body. He had amazing testimonials, including Howard Stern.

Up until that point, I was about 10 years deep into my mindfulness training journey, but It wasn't for healing, it was for inner peace. Then it dawned on me that it could be the same thing. I researched more and found Dr. Joe Dispenza. He also had amazing testimonies of healings just from teaching people how to meditate and visualize. It made sense, the brain is attached to the spine which then has nerves that go out to the entire body.

One day, I was on the floor doing my postural therapy and a major divine download hit me. "Put all 3 methods together and make it ONE!"

I jumped up off the floor and started pacing in my living room.

The next download came: "Open a virtual clinic, you don't have to touch anyone."

Whoa.

The next download came: "Put the body back into full alignment and the body will do its own work."

Brilliant!

This would be the birth of my book, PEACE OVER PAIN along with the PEACE OVER PAIN Virtual Clinic.

The concept was simple.

Your body is a vehicle. The structure of that vehicle is the musculoskeletal system. Now the vehicle needs fuel. That fuel is the nutrition. And inside the vehicle is an onboard computer called the mind that controls everything. BOOM! Easy to understand.

My theory was that all 3 methods needed to be practiced at the same time to put the body into a state of healing. This state of healing would work for EVERY chronic condition someone was not born with.

During school for postural therapy, I learned how to evaluate bodies. It was a method of looking at photos of bodies from the front, back, and both sides. Doing this, a trained eye could notice misalignments. The school had their own software but it was limited and more AI generated. I decided to go rogue and view my photos in a different program on my computer.

While I was practicing looking at posture photos (p-rays) I figured out how to make straight lines and zoom in close. This gave me a whole new perspective of the body. I could zoom in on the feet and notice hammer toes, bunions, flat feet etcetera. I could zoom in on the spine and see bulging discs and humps.

Then I added nutrition and mental health to the intake forms of the client. Now I was able to connect dots at a level no one had ever seen before. Could this person's migraines be coming from their forward head posture, their nutritional deficiencies or their mind? Hmm. Guess what!? It doesn't matter because my new method would work for all 3 at the same time.

Then I screen captured me doing this evaluation and I would send the client a link to the video. People were shocked. I invented something brand new that was more thorough than blood labs or x-rays because it shows the entire body and how it all connects.

I found a way to evaluate the whole body whereas the Medical Monopoly just looks at the body through the eyes of speciality. Then, they treat the symptoms instead of going after the entire body. Not us, we actually count the symptoms. That's right, you leave your analysis with a symptoms score and that gives you a gauge as to what direction you're going in.

So for example, if you scored a 30 on your analysis and your score in a few months is a 15, you're moving in the right direction. You're healing. If you don't do anything, your symptoms will increase because that's just common sense as you age.

This evaluation helps you find the root causes of your symptoms and even more importantly, it gives you the "ah-ha" moment you need to understand my new health approach.

In November of 2022, I ended up going viral on Instagram and soon an audience formed. My DMs filled up with people that needed help and I was in a position to help them.

Over the course of the next year, we collected so many testimonies on camera from people all over the world. They were healing everything from frozen shoulders, herniated disks, sciatica, type 2 diabetes, neuropathy, scoliosis, PCOS and so much more. The system worked. The divine downloads were correct.

Unfortunately, it wasn't too long before attacks on me started. I noticed that what really got people triggered was that I had a PhD and not a MD. Therefore, I was called a quack, a snake oil salesman and a grifter. After a few months of the bashings (and death threats), I would proclaim myself to be a FAKE DOCTOR with REAL RESULTS.

To the haters, debaters and vigilantes, It didn't matter that I had all these testimonies on video, they didn't care. I realized that I needed to stop calling myself a "holistic doctor" in order to protect myself. I began to refer to myself as a healer instead. The term doctor was now just part of my "stage name" since I could actually use it with my PhD.

One day I was talking to one of my staff members (Tamra) and I said something along the lines of, "Yea, we gotta heal them from head to toe." BOOM. A light bulb went off. HEAD TO TOE HEALING. That's it! That's what this new method should be called. She didn't like it, but I stayed firm with my idea. I just knew it was going to catch on.

I felt that HEAD TO TOE HEALING described this new health approach so well because we are going after the whole body and because of that, it didn't matter what condition the person was diagnosed with.

HEAD TO TOE HEALING became the answer to everything...

Question: "Dr. Reese, what do I do about my fibromyalgia?"

Answer: HEAD TO TOE HEALING

Question: "Dr. Reese, what do I do about my herniated disk?"

Answer: HEAD TO TOE HEALING

Question: "Dr. Reese, what do I do about my type 2 diabetes?"

Answer: HEAD TO TOE HEALING

I started to call myself the only HEAD TO TOE HEALER in the world. Some people would get triggered and say, "Barbra O'Neil, Dr. Berg and Dr. Sebi are head to toe healers too." And I would respond, "What would they do with a herniated disk or a bunion? Sprinkle herbs on it?"

I had something new going on here whether they wanted to open their eyes to it or not.

Soon, I wrote 2 more books. Reverse The Cause which detailed the root causes of 60+ chronic conditions. My goal was to open people's eyes as to how HEAD TO TOE HEALING works and how there can be so many causes involved with your conditions. Then I wrote DINNER W/ DR. REESE which was a unique cookbook with 100 recipes that were "poor 4 free." I wanted to show that you can eat really well without these 4 foods.

One day I was talking to a doctor mentor of mine and he suggested that I was "playing with fire." He said that my HEAD TO TOE analysis acted as a diagnosis and the supplements and protocols we were giving our clients acted as "medicine." He said the courts would view it as "practicing without a license" even though I technically wasn't. I had to make a big decision, especially with all the attacks coming my way. Doctors were now bashing me on social media and calling me dangerous.

As the attacks on me grew, it was a smart idea to shut down my virtual clinic and start a virtual learning membership instead. My company took a major financial hit. We went from charging $8200 per client to

$55/mo for members. This was a huge risk because now we were relying on volume to stay alive. The company struggled for months.

I focused my attention on this membership like my life depended on it. My goal was to over deliver in the membership. This may have backfired a little because it just made it a little overwhelming. After about 4 months, I realized that the star of the show was the live classes, the HEAD TO TOE HEALING 120 challenge and having access to the best supplements in the world. So we started to focus on these 3 features.

The membership was more "school-like" and gave us an opportunity to TEACH more people the practice of HEAD TO TOE HEALING instead of taking one on one clients. This got us out of that "practicing without a license" danger zone. The membership was educational. We simply supplied people with classes, courses and community.

I continued to do my livestream on Tuesdays at 6pm Est and we added in a members zoom room. It wasn't long before members would talk on the livestream and give their testimonies of their healing results. We started collecting testimonials on video at an amazing rate from people all over the world like Japan, the UK, Australia, New Zealand, Nigeria and more. Symptoms were disappearing.

The craziest part was I've never met with, sat down with or even knew their names. They simply enter the membership and follow the teachings of HEAD TO TOE HEALING and it miraculously works. It's a system. I'm actually not needed at all!

At the current time, it's obvious that we have the most healing results ever recorded on video. It's all due to this new practice that I created called HEAD TO TOE HEALING. This is so important because it proves that you can live pain and drug-free and unplug from the Medical Monopoly.

In this green book I would like to show you the testimonials in written form. Of course the videos are all on my website:

www.DRKEVINREESE.com but sometimes reading them can be more profound.

If you wish to wake someone up that is stuck in a medical prison, I suggest giving them the red book (Medical Monopoly) as well as this green book (Head To Toe Healing).

Allow the red and green to do its work.

Thank you, I love you.

14-Hour Long Gallbladder Pain Completely Gone

Dr. Reese:

You did the program. Okay, so what's the story? How did that start?

Woman:

It started in December. Before that, I probably didn't even know what a gallstone was or where it was in my body. I'd never even heard of it or paid attention to it. Then I realized the pain I was experiencing was gallstone pain—it started at the end of December. As soon as I realized I was having gallstone pain, I started searching through your videos and comments to try to find anything gallstone-related. There was a comment on Instagram that said you had just come out with a gallstone course. So, I signed up for that—I was like, sign me up that night!

I was so excited when the course came through. I made notes on everything—what to do, my new protocol—and I've been following it. I haven't had an attack since. So many people were quick to tell me to go and get my gallbladder out the next day. When I posted on Facebook, as soon as I realized I was having gallstones, 90% of the comments were, "Go get surgery, go get surgery." But I didn't want that. I've never believed in the medical monopoly.

So, I was looking for ways to heal it myself, and I was so glad to have your course. I haven't had an attack since. I used to get them once or twice a month since December, when this new thing happened to me. I'm still in the beginning stages of healing it, but I haven't had any problems yet. I'm very excited about that.

So many people are asking about it. There are all these gallstone groups on Facebook, and I've been tagging your pages. I'm like, "Listen, do this, follow this." Hopefully, some of them will listen too.

Dr. Reese:

Yeah. Well, I appreciate you sharing your story. That's really great to hear. You know, that's why I put it out there. So many people are under attack with their gallbladders. And people aren't just going to randomly come to our main program. That's a big program—it's thousands and thousands of dollars. It's a whole year. I mean, it's a big deal. Yet, there are all these people whose gallbladders are on the verge of being taken out.

I needed to find a way to support those people who just need to flip it around real quick. Just real quick, right? I believe in the video I said, "Look, this is immediate. This is urgent. You've got to change things right now." And it sounds like you followed that perfectly.

Woman:

Yeah, and it was urgent because the pain was worse than labor pains. It was worse than any pain I could describe. I couldn't even be on my phone—I couldn't even scroll through social media or function when I was in a gallstone attack. They lasted an average of six hours, and my last one was 14 hours. I couldn't sleep, couldn't touch my phone, couldn't do anything but be in absolute agony. That's why people were telling me, "Just go rip it out, rip it out."

Dr. Reese:

Fourteen hours of pain?

Woman:

That was my last one. The average was six to seven hours. When it got close to the six-hour mark, I'd think, "All right, we're almost done," but then it just kept going.

Dr. Reese:

And no more attacks? That's awesome.

Woman:

I haven't had one since I've done the program. I bought all three books and loved reading them. I couldn't put the first book down! I'm not even a big reader, but I gave it to my family to read. Now I have the cookbook and the other book, and I'm all about healing my body naturally. I feel better, and I didn't have to go through surgery for that.

Dr. Reese:

That's awesome. Thank you for sharing that.

Woman:

Yeah, thank you for your knowledge. It helped me solve this big problem of mine.

Dr. Reese:

You're very welcome.

Bulging Discs Gone, Frozen Shoulder Gone & Immobility Gone

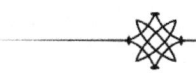

"The reason why I joined the program and started following Kevin in the first place was because I was having bulging discs in the back of my neck and they were creating a pinched nerve down my right arm that was very severe and very painful and was really just doing horrible things to my quality of life. I was having trouble with simple mobility, I couldn't wear certain clothes because I couldn't get in and out of them, my daily life was completely interrupted by the lack of mobility and just really by the pain.

I just want to say the pain itself was gone within three weeks which was just completely incredible to me. I had no idea that it would work that fast. After the issues that I was having with my arm and not moving it for several months because of the pain, I also got a frozen shoulder. I was just able to work through the frozen shoulder in a way that I was not able to do before that. And within, I would say, maybe two months, the mobility that I had in my arm was completely different than when I entered the program. Meaning I could wash my hair with both hands, I can put my hair up in a ponytail again, I can wear any of the clothes in my closet, I don't have to think about if it's a button front or what do I wear underneath it before getting dressed every single day.

It's just changed my life completely and I can't thank all of you enough. I appreciate each and every one of you and Kevin especially. I just appreciate you dedicating your life to helping others and to doing it in a way that's easy to watch.

You really prepare people, I think, for the program and what it will be like. And then your team just jumps in and makes sure we follow it and that we get what we need to get done and answer any questions. And I'm thrilled.

I am so thrilled. I am exactly where I hoped I would be at the end of the program. And I know that I'll have all of you around for several

Costochondritis Gone, Plantar Fasciitis Gone, Numbness in Legs Gone, Cracked Heels Gone, Age Spots Disappearing

"So for 30 years I've had inhalers, multiple inhalers for my asthma.

An asthma attack feels like I'm going to stop breathing. My chest is so tight, it feels so heavy, like my lungs are just going to give out on me. It's not a good feeling.

Never for one minute did I think changing the way I eat would have anything to do with my asthma, making it better. I no longer have to use any of my inhalers. I no longer have asthma attacks. I feel so much better. My allergies to pets are much better. They don't trigger my asthma.

My eyes don't start burning or itching. My skin doesn't start swelling up anymore. I've also had eczema for about 18 years now and since doing the program I haven't had any eczema outbreaks at all. I'm shocked that all these results happened. I feel so much better."

ASTHMA GONE, ALLERGIES GONE AND ECZEMA GONE

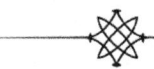

months to come to coach me through, you know, the next steps and all of that as I continue to recover from the frozen shoulder.

But again, thank you so much. I am speechless. I'm so happy and I want to thank all of you."

LISA: I've made some progress with the numbing in my legs, which is huge for me, because when we first met, when I would bend my legs, I felt like the skin was going to crack and pop in half. They were so tight. I don't have the numbing anymore.

COACH SHAWN: As far as her numbers, her blood sugar score went from a 2 to a 0. Her soft tissue went from a 6 to a 2.5. Her hard tissue went from a 6 to a 2. Brittle hair is getting a lot better. Her age spots are starting to disappear. Grey hair is improving immensely. No more cracked heels. The numbness has gone away. Plantar fasciitis is gone, which is a big one. And her hip pain is gone. So she's definitely making a lot of progress.

COACH SHAWN: And her posture looks really good.

DR. REESE: Lisa, you've made a ton of progress. There's no more plantar fasciitis?

LISA: I have. It was huge. And honestly, one day I was like, oh, my God, I don't feel my plantar anymore. I really couldn't tell you when it happened. It just happened. I'm like, this is amazing since it's so debilitating for me as a dog walker.

COACH SHAWN: That's awesome. That's great. Yeah. You went from 20 symptoms to 9 symptoms Lisa.

LISA: Yay! Also, no more costochondritis. I haven't had that at all since I've been on your program.

DR. REESE: That's amazing. That's great.

LISA: Yeah. I haven't been sick at all since I've done your program.

Insomnia Gone

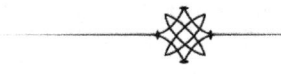

DR. REESE: So you're sleeping better, huh?

ANDREA: Oh yeah, that's great. I'm so impressed.

DR. REESE: How bad was the insomnia before?

ANDREA: I went years with hardly getting any sleep. Maybe six years, I was hardly, like maybe getting four hours a night. It was horrible and it just ruined my health. And gosh, this is the best I've come across.

I used to take all kinds of holistic stuff, patches, you know, I've done protocols before and had other naturopaths and stuff.

DR. REESE: Very cool. I'm really glad to hear that. Thank you for sharing.

HIP PAIN GONE IN 2 WEEKS

DR. REESE: So Ed, you're dancing again, your pain is gone?

EDWARD: Yes, it's amazing. You know, I just finished up my 120 this past week and you know, I can't say enough about the whole program.

I was having trouble dancing. We travel a lot, my wife and I do. And we have these conferences and sometimes on Saturday night they'll have a two-hour dance.

And before the program I could only dance maybe, you know, one long country song until my hips were hurting so bad I couldn't wait for the song to be over with. And we just had another conference a little over a month ago and it was a two-hour long deal and I danced for two hours, never stopped. Even my wife got tired and had to go sit down for a minute and I still stayed out there dancing.

DR. REESE: Wow.

EDWARD: The reason I got started in the program in the first place was my hip, my hips were hurting, my knee was hurting, I was having really bad back pain when I would go to bed trying to turn or toss, it would just hurt so bad it would take my breath away. And, you know, all of that went away within two weeks. And it just, you know, it rocks. It's awesome, man.

DR. REESE: It's so good to hear.

Psoriasis Gone in 30 Days

DR. REESE: Mitch has been on the program for under 30 days and he had psoriasis and he no longer is itchy or inflamed and his skin looks great.

MITCH: I know. It's going good and I'm starting to come out on the other end. Now, the first couple of weeks, just getting into a routine was a little bit challenging, but once you've got it down, I'm telling Karen and she's been a great support network for me. And yeah, I'm feeling good. Always had a problem and I just kind of started narrowing it down and then, yeah, I found you.

DR. REESE: That's pretty cool.

MITCH: It's under 30 days. I'm looking fantastic and my sleep's better. Everything's better.

DR. REESE: That's great to hear, man.

PCOS, Diabetes, Gut Issues, Body Pain & Duck Feet Gone

LEAH: So coming into this I have PCOS which is polycystic ovarian syndrome and that comes with everything from skin issues, excess hair growth, fatigue. I would never get a period. Years and years would go by and I'd maybe get one every two to three years. On this program alone, the four months I've been on it, I've gotten a period every month. And that's unheard of with my health.

With PCOS you have insulin resistance and I did have type 2 diabetes so my sugar levels would be in the 200s pretty regularly. And on this program, they've been in the low 100s over the past four months which is just giving me more energy. I'm not having super crazy cravings for anything. I sleep better because my sugar isn't so elevated. I'd have a tough time with number twos, and just feeling bloated all the time and nothing seemed to agree with my stomach. It was hard to pinpoint what the issue was. I have lost 30 pounds on the program. And now my number twos are great.

So that's definitely improved on this program and again it's only been four months so just imagine in another eight months, you know, a full year doing this how good you could feel and I'm already feeling so much better.

Also, I had everything from knee pain, joint pain, back pain, hip pain, just overall tightness and just feeling very slouchy. And with the postural therapy and the program, I don't even think about knee pain. I don't feel it. My hips don't have any achiness or tightness anymore. I used to walk like a duck, like my feet were pointed out and now with the program and the postural therapy my feet are so much straighter and that's just helping my gait and how I walk and I'm sure my hips and my joints, and everything are more in alignment which is amazing.

I definitely have more flexibility, more stamina, and just overall feeling so much better.

Interview with Leah

JOE: So with me tonight, I have Leah. Now, what do you do for a living? What have you done as a career, occupation?

LEAH: Yeah, so I'm a little all over the place. I work a full-time job at a desk—kind of administrative customer service-type work. Pretty much my whole working life has been at a desk, five days a week, eight hours a day, so I'm sitting a lot. But on the flip side of that, I also work in a restaurant in the kitchen part-time. So when I'm working there, I'm on my feet, lifting things, crouching, crawling, doing all the things that you do in a kitchen.

JOE: So, when did you first start having medical issues? When was your first inkling that you needed to see a doctor for something that possibly happened on the job or otherwise?

LEAH: Well, I have a condition called PCOS, which is polycystic ovarian syndrome. I've had that since puberty—basically for 20 or more years, at this point probably 25 years. That's when things started to feel off in my body, and I started going to gynecologists and doctors. I was an overweight kid at the time, and while weight doesn't cause the condition, it is part of it. It's harder to lose weight, and you gain weight easily. Anytime I went to a doctor, it was always the same: "Lose weight, take this pill, see me in six months." But it never did anything for me. If anything, the pills I took made me feel worse or created new issues that then required another pill to fix.

LEAH: Outside of that condition, PCOS also causes insulin resistance, and I developed diabetes. And that comes with a slew of its own issues—fatigue, sugar fluctuations, eyesight problems, and risks to your heart, kidneys, and other organs. A lot of people in my family have gone down the diabetes and heart disease road. Over the past 10 years, I started seeing the same pattern happening to me. I would try to take care of it, watch what I ate, adjust my diet, but nothing ever stuck. Then this past year, I was like, I *have* to do something. My sugar levels were crazy, my body aches were ridiculous, and I just felt drained and tired all the time.

JOE: Your quality of life wasn't where you wanted it to be—it was pretty low at that point, right?

LEAH: Exactly. So for me, it was a question of: Do I want to go down the road I've seen others go down, knowing the end result? Or do I want to take control and make a change for the rest of my life?

JOE: Well, you had been going to the medical monopoly for years, right? And it started with one condition that became chronic because all they did was slap a Band-Aid on it. "Lose weight, take this pill, come back in six months." You came back, and the issue was still there. Maybe a little smaller, maybe a little different, but it was still there. And over time, instead of improving, it snowballed into diabetes, heart concerns, weight issues, and a declining quality of life.

JOE: So what made you decide to break away from the medical monopoly? You had the option to continue down that road. What was the deciding factor that made you say, "That's it. No more. I'm taking my health into my own hands"?

LEAH: I think most people initially trust the medical system because it's what we've been given. We're told, "Go to a doctor; they know what they're doing. They'll help you." And you can't blame people for thinking that because it's what we've been conditioned to believe. But after seeing my family go down the road of heart surgeries, kidney dialysis, and never getting better, I realized I needed an alternative.

LEAH: I also realized that doctors don't have real conversations with you anymore. They type things into a computer, follow a list of questions, and then prescribe something. There's no support. No one ever suggested lifestyle changes—nutrition, mindfulness, posture. It was always about treating symptoms instead of addressing root causes.

JOE: Right. They follow protocols. "Here's your prescription; see you in six months."

LEAH: Exactly. And when I saw my family stuck in that system, I knew I needed to find something different. That's when I started looking into alternatives, and I came across Dr. Reese—through you, actually!

JOE: Oh wow.

LEAH: Yeah, following your social media, and then through algorithms, more natural health solutions started popping up. I found Dr. Reese's podcasts, read his testimonials, got his book, and everything he said just made sense. It wasn't radical—it was logical.

JOE: And now, six months in, your PCOS is regulated, your diabetes has improved, and you're off the medical monopoly treadmill.

LEAH: Yes! And I haven't needed to go back.

FROZEN SHOULDER GONE & DEPRESSION GONE

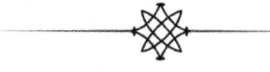

LORRAINE: I can do the Matrix now!

DR. REESE: I just want everyone to know that she couldn't lift her arms up, what, three months ago?

LORRAINE: I couldn't move my right arm at all. And now I can. I'm very blessed to have come across all your paths and my coach Keysha is phenomenal.

DR. REESE: Good, good. I just wanted to bring you on at this moment so that someone like Susie can see where she's gonna be in a few months. Cause you, you are, you know, what we like to call a hot mess.

LORRAINE: I couldn't do a lot of exercise, so I was immobile. And I think I had, well, I know I had depression and then, you know, got off the floor and with the nutrition supplements like I have my energy back.

LORRAINE: I started bike riding eight miles a day last week. It's just been a total reverse. And now it is just like, I don't want anything interfering with that and the supplements just let me feel good and to be present.

LORRAINE: I feel good to just have all my nutrition and I'm so happy.

DR. REESE: Good, good. Well, I tell your story all the time that you couldn't wash your hair and then you finally could wash your hair.

LORRAINE: Thank you Dr. Reese.

Gray hair and Age Spots Gone?

WOMAN: "One minute I wasn't feeling right and the next minute I found Dr. Reese on Instagram. That's how it happened. I mean yeah, I really don't know how this happened.

I'm the one with the gray hair and I no longer have gray hair.

COACH TAMRA: I was just noticing your hair wow! It's really dark, look at that!

WOMAN: My husband said to me, "your eyebrows, they're so dark." I don't know where, but it's wild.

LEVI: Did you have a lot of gray hair or was it like on the roots?

WOMAN: The roots, so it was often I have to dye it like every three, four weeks. Now it's been months. My hair got darker. I was like, wow. I also had quite a few age spots on my hands and arms. Now I have maybe a little bit on one hand. That's it. Get on these nutrients and there you go.

DR. REESE: Is that Joan that I saw? Our favorite non-gray-haired person? Our dark brunette. Oh, look at that.

WOMAN: It's a good thing. And I was telling them I had age spots, quite a few. Now I have just a few, which is good. It's pretty cool.

DR. REESE: You're reversing in age. You're going to be 20 in a second.

WOMAN: I know. It's scary. Very scary.

Hot Flashes Eliminated, Feet Pain Gone, Back Pain Gone, and Sleep Restored

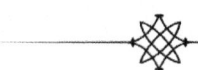

DR. REESE: What was life like with the pain?

HILLARY: Just getting up in the morning, you always felt like you couldn't. Like getting out of bed just hurts. So you shuffle, you know.

But now it's like I can get out of bed, I bounce out of bed and do my little affirmations and feel, you know, just start the day in a different way. I still do my cats and dogs just to make sure I get all the kinks out, but still, I don't get out of bed with the foot pain and the back pain or get out of bed because I was sweating.

DR. REESE: How does that change your sleeping?

HILLARY: When I wake up in the morning, I'm like, oh my gosh, I didn't wake up, you know, so the things that you don't think about now is what, oh shoot, that's gone, you know, like I didn't think about my back pain, I didn't think about the night sweats because they're not there. And then I realized, oh shoot, it's so nice because it's just kind of out of sight, out of mind. And then when Karen's like, well, how's this? I'm like, oh, that's right. I don't have it. I don't have it. So it's wonderful.

SCIATICA PAIN GONE IN 70 DAYS

GLEN: Yeah, it was about two weeks ago. And all of a sudden the stabbing, killing, chronic burning pain just got less. And I was kind of surprised because I didn't believe it, but out of the blue, it started to diminish. I must say, things have gotten better. I just flew down here into the Bahamas today. I can tell you that the last time I flew down here and flew back, I could not sit in the chair.

I was in so much agony. It was horrible. The last two weekends I've been essentially from a 20 to a 10 and maybe to a 1 or 2 in the pain department and there's no explanation for that other than what I'm doing. The pain that I have now is not debilitating. It does not put me on the floor every minute of the day that I'm not working. So kudos to you and your team and all that you've recommended.

To anyone that is not so sure, this is your guy. Because if you get trapped in the medical monopoly, you're done. It's just a matter of time before they kill you. They will kill you with whatever poison they give you, whatever test, whatever radiation, chemo, whatever, you're done.

DR. REESE: I appreciate you coming on here.

GLEN: Thank you for all you do. Dr. Reese, anybody out there, I'm telling you, this is your guy. If you've got any problems, get away from the medical mafia do yourself right and see Dr. Reese.

COACH SHAWN: We appreciate you, Dr. G.

GLEN: And I appreciate you guys a lot. Thank you for saving me

GLEN: I had all kinds of things going on my body, like my chest was sticking out and I had a hernia down low. And, you know, no one ever had an explanation. "Oh, you got a small hernia, you got this, you got that." But we're almost 11 months into the membership program now, and this hernia that I had is pretty much gone.

DR. REESE: Wow.

GLEN: Just, you know, it was below my belly button, just right in the center, and now it's almost flat. There it is. No pills, no lotions, no potions, no surgery, no drugs. Just doing your head-to-toe healing work. That's it. It has more implications than you think. Because you would never think that that's a big thing, but then all of a sudden it disappears and I just had my eyes checked at the medical machine over there and my eye pressure is down. And they were scratching their head because they're waiting to, they keep trying to sell me surgery for my eyes and I'm like, no. And I'm like, aren't you curious why my eye pressure is down without THC or something like that?

Tinnitus Gone, Vertigo Gone, Jaw Clicking Gone, IBS Gone and Ear Unblocked

DR. REESE: So you had a blocked ear?

ANGELA: Yes, so the left ear had been blocking up for over a couple of years now, and I've had it off and on. Always had problems with that left ear blocking and had to get it cleaned out. The clicking jaw, I've had that forever, since childhood probably. And that's all gone as well. So these things just started disappearing one at a time. The ringing in my ear and the dizziness were gone. The biggest issue for me too at the moment was the IBS and that was the first to go.

DR. REESE: Wow, well done, wow.

ANGELA: I'm like grinning like a Cheshire cat, I can't stop. The physio and the hospital orthopedics said they can't believe how I've healed up so quickly like a 30 year old, you know I'm like an old lady 62.

DR. REESE: That gray hair is gonna go away too.

ANGELA: It's already starting, you can see it. it was white you know and now It's changing color. It's unreal.

DR. REESE: Yeah, I'm super happy for you. This is what we do it for.

ANGELA: You've joined all the dots. Out of every other doctor, you've connected the whole thing together. And I knew that immediately. And it's logical, because I'm one of those annoying patients that say to doctors, "but why? Why have I got this? What's caused it?", And they go, "oh sorry it's genetic." Yeah. Really? That's what they do to you and they just fob you off. "Oh the pill stopped working after two months that you put me on for this. Oh well it's alright because we got a new one out you can try that." You just go round the merry-go-round and you don't get better. Yeah. Yeah, so that's the way it's worked for me. That's why I'm here.

DR. REESE: Thank you for sharing with us. That was great.

Acid Reflux Gone, Knee Pain Gone, Migraines Gone, Baldness Gone, Brain Fog Gone, and Grew Half Of An Inch!?

DR. REESE: What about your knee pain?

JANET: Knee pain! The inflammation went down so much when I stopped the oil. I spend a lot of time kneeling on my prayers. I got through three rosaries today. I was okay,

DR. REESE: So your knee pain is gone, what about heartburn?

JANET: Yeah, I haven't had heartburn. I would just bend down to pick up my dog and then I'd get the acid throat.

DR. REESE: And you don't get that anymore?

JANET: It's been five months I'd say.

DR. REESE: That's really nice. I've had that. And how about your nails?

JANET: Nails have almost no more ridges. Also, I used to get three-day migraines every month. They're all gone.

DR. REESE: Congratulations.

DR. REESE: What other improvements have you had?

JANET: My hair. Well, I just blow-dried it now, but I have baldness in this area. I used to make my bangs, like, come from here, just to look thicker. It's growing much faster. I just feel good all over, but my brain fog stopped In three weeks. It just went away. We had it really bad right I could feel my brain fuzzy all day long.

DR. REESE: Tell us how you're feeling.

JANET: I'm feeling wonderful. I got a half inch back.

DR. REESE: You grew a half inch?

JANET: I did, I'm not so 90 year old anymore. But I was a caregiver for many years, so I was always in the hunched position lifting. So I just became that shape 24 hours a day.

"I used to get really debilitating migraines, like bad. And now I'm not laid up hiding in hibernation. The sign that everything would be up here because it triggers the sinus infections, everything is all connected. Now I feel like everything is moving. And Coach Connor is awesome.

Like he's got me working. I can see it. And then I lost, I mean, I wasn't trying to lose all this weight, but you know when you eliminate stuff and when your digestive is on point, I lost 10 pounds.

I just feel light as a feather, like I feel so much lighter. It's amazing.

So thank you very much."

Hashimoto's Symptoms Reduced and Knee Pain Gone

"I've had pretty severe Hashimoto's for 13 years. And in the last 13 years, I have not had two days in a row without some kind of moderate to severe symptom. So literally not two days in a row symptom-free and also not two days in a row with good sleep.

I would say my symptoms were around probably 85% of the time. Now, my symptoms are around 30% of the time.

That's amazing to me. You know, like that alone is a really good start. And I've always been somewhat athletic, but because of the inflammation, I couldn't get up and down off the ground without a lot of trouble with my knees.

My wife and I go walking probably four or five times a week, and I could never run. I can run a little bit now which makes her laugh so much because she's like, you look so funny because you haven't been running in so long."

"So much stuff is healed, as you know. Like my shoulders and knees were killing me before and now they're not bothering me. My eyesight was freaked out, ringing my ears. I mean, so many different things.

And the cost of the membership, I mean, the cost of the whole thing, everything, that's worth its weight in gold right there. So thank you guys. And I love you."

Fibroids Gone, Psoriasis Gone and Migraines Gone

"I was in pain from having painful periods, migraines, and I was having psoriasis issues. And for whatever reason, all of that was happening all at the same time. And so I just put it out there on Facebook because I was so frustrated that all of this was happening to me. So I just said, I'm in a lot of pain, and I can't take this anymore. Kevin came in on my status and stated to me, what are you going through?

So I inboxed Kevin and told him everything that I was going through with my psoriasis, my migraines, my painful periods, and the constant bleeding, me having to call out of work and stuff, and the doctor stating that I possibly needing surgery to get rid of my fibroids, either removing the fibroids or removing my uterus. Kevin says, "you do not have to do this. You don't have to have the surgery. You don't have to go through this. Why don't you come and work with me?"

Within 30 days, my migraines were gone. 30 days after that, my psoriasis was gone. It was a few months, about 90 days, when the fibroids started to shrink. And at my follow-up appointment with my doctor at that time, one of the fibroids that was the size of a grapefruit was the size of a lemon, and the two that were a size of a lemon were now tiny peanut sizes.

And the bleeding had started getting less and less. And the amount of days that I was on my periods, they were shortened. I was on a regular schedule. The painful fibroids went away. I definitely became a believer in the program. I believe in the program so much I'm out there telling other people about it. I'm constantly promoting it."

"I went to the doctors probably like 90 days later, like 90 days in the program, And she had stated that, "Oh, your fibrase have shrunk". The one that was the size of a grapefruit shrunk down to the size of a lemon.

And the two that were the size of lemons shrunk down to size of grapes. My migraines are gone in 30 days."

Off Blood Pressure Meds and Hormone Replacement Therapy (HRT)

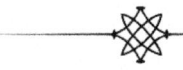

DR. REESE: Maria, you're off your blood pressure medication now?

MARIA: 100%

DR. REESE: Wow.

MARIA: And off the HRTs.

DR. REESE: HRTs gone. Wow. Finally.

MARIA: I'm completely off of everything and could not be happier.

DR. REESE: That was a big deal for you coming into the program. I remember.

MARIA: Oh, I mean, it was a huge deal. I mean, that was probably the primary motivator for me to get off all of the medications. And it took a while, right? As you always say, not everybody has results in, you know, the first two weeks. Good six months.

MARIA: I've told Shawn. I've told Karen, that there is not a day that goes by that I do not give thanks for you and your team. I am so grateful that I found you guys because it's amazing. This literally is life-altering. I was headed down a really scary path, you know, with all of the synthetic meds that I was on.

DR. REESE: How was your gut on day one versus day 120?

MARIA: So initially it was just a mixture of constipation, diarrhea, just a general sad tummy. And now the only time I have an issue is when I either knowingly cheat or unknowingly get something in my system that I'm no longer accustomed to, you know, mostly the gluten and then my tummy lets me know that you've been a bad girl but I mean if I don't fall off the wagon I feel great.

DR. REESE: I mean look how skinny you are!

No More Walking Cane!

DR. REESE: So you used to walk with a cane, but you're not right now?

MAN: Well, about a year ago I had a severe arthritis hip pain really bad. And I was using a stick, yeah. And it gives you the motivation to stay off that gluten, to stay off, you know, when you go out and you see gluten stuff and junk food everywhere, to have people around to help you, you know, because I've got my family saying, "go and get it done, get your hip done, blah, blah, blah". But I keep telling them "who wants to do that?" This is the support you get.

MAN: I've signed up for other memberships before and you just get a manual. To have live therapy and people to call and people to speak to and listen to, It's just fantastic and I'm very thankful for it because it's just fun.

DR. REESE: That's great to hear. Thank you so much for sharing with us. You're just going to keep getting better too.

MAN: This membership is just so much fun. What can I say?

Numbness Gone, Raynaud's Gone, Irregular Heartbeat Gone in 60 Days. No more Neck Brace or ER Visits

CLERIL: I've experienced so many benefits so far, as opposed to running to the hospital, maybe what, two, three times a month with no progress whatsoever. Indeed, the numbness is gone, the coldness is gone, but I've been so much better in just sixty days. I can remember the first time I had my video with Amber. I could have barely, you know, I could have barely talked really. I was so weak. I was tired. Now I am more energetic than ever.

DR. REESE: That's good news, man. You're only halfway there, correct?

CLERIL: I got a long way to go, but, you know, it's been great so far. I understand a lot of people might have some skepticism. I get it. There's a lot of people out here fooling folks but I can say for certain this is not a joke. This is not a scam. It is real because it really helped me and is helping me.

DR. REESE: Very cool. I appreciate those words.

Kidney function restored. Chronic constipation, astigmatism, and nodules gone. All blood tests improved drastically.

LINDA: I can sleep very well, I don't wake up from any kind of pain in my body or anything like that. I don't know where I would be today if Bill had not given me Dr. Reese's book. And he found it because he was trying to help me not cry anymore. Because I was... In that much pain. Pretty bad, yeah."

"You know, Dr. Reese, for a good 50, 60 years, I've always been constipated and really bad. I mean, I would go weeks and never have a bowel movement. I mean, it was crazy.

And finally, you and I finally figured out, you put me on that cleanse and Hallelujah, Halle-back. I can't believe it. I'm sitting there saying to myself, how long has it been in there?"

DR. REESE: What did you tell the eye doctor?

LINDA: Well, I was more asking questions to her why I've always just had it, but I have an astigmatism in my left eye. And I've had a prescription that would, you know, make that astigmatism not blurry, just getting worse. So when she told me that my prescription had changed I said ,"okay".

So you know what happened? She said ,"Well your astigmatism is getting better."

I go, "what do you mean by that? So explain that to me because what do you mean it's three times better?"

She had to change my prescription up to three times better than what it was. So I was like so blurry because my eye was better and it was trying to look through blur. I was trying to look too old, you know, where it was when it was not better.

My eye doctor goes, "what do you do?" And I said, "well, I take a lot of supplements and I'm in a program."

DR. REESE: Yeah, you're hanging around a charlatan with a rabbit.

LINDA: That's right. So that's how I see this program is my Fountain of Youth.

LINDA: I had these nodules on my head up here and I had one inside here in my gum and this one in my gum just disappeared. My doctor wanted to do surgery and I happened to start with Dr. Reese.

And so when my dentist said, "So why don't you come in and we'll take that", I said, "I'm okay. I'm good. I've got it fixed."

DR. REESE: It's a lifestyle surgery, you know.

LINDA: It is. It was wonderful. It was so nice to tell him, I don't need him and it's gone.

DR. REESE: Fire him! Fire him!

LINDA: I did fire him! It was right then and there. The one on my forehead it's still there but it's getting smaller. I can't wait for another four months.

Interview with Linda

JOE: Welcome, everybody, we are actually going to talk to one of our clients and find out about Linda Troutman's story. Linda, how are you?

JOE: What did you do for a living out there when you were working?

LINDA: Well, when I first started my life, I was married at 19.

JOE: Yes, that's the way it was in our day.

LINDA: Yeah, my mom got married at 21.

JOE: Yeah.

LINDA: We were raised to get married, have kids, and all that stuff, you know? So, I got my beauty license and became a hairdresser. I worked for two years and then got pregnant. It's just the next thing that happens when you get married young, right?

JOE: Right.

LINDA: I went back to work for two weeks and decided to quit because I wanted to raise my child myself. Every time I called the daycare, she was crying, didn't like it. So, I quit being a hairdresser and became a stay-at-home mom. But I knew I had to work, so I became a daycare provider. My girlfriend—well, it was fabulous. It really was. It was the thing I was supposed to do. I ended up doing that for 40 years.

JOE: Oh, okay. So, you were a daycare provider, worked with kids for 40 years?

LINDA: Yeah.

JOE: That's a lot of running around, right?

LINDA: Yes.

JOE: That must have been taxing on the body. Kids on the back, kids on the front, kids on the hips.

LINDA: Yes. I carried four or five kids around all the time.

JOE: Right. Plus, you had your own at home. How many do you have?

LINDA: I have three daughters. But today, I have my three daughters and two stepdaughters. So, Bill and I have five girls.

JOE: Five girls.

LINDA: Yep.

JOE: That's fun.

LINDA: Eleven grandchildren and four great-grandchildren.

JOE: Wow, Linda. You've got quite a family tree going on there.

LINDA: Yep.

JOE: You've definitely done your duty.

LINDA: And they're all out of my house.

JOE: Well, that's a good thing. So, right now, are you retired? Just chilling up there in San Jose?

LINDA: No, actually not. Bill and I both work a security job. He's in security, and I'm in security. I take care of Amazon and Apple buildings.

JOE: You put on the uniform?

LINDA: I do. Every day.

JOE: Wow, well, good for you.

LINDA: Yeah.

JOE: I hope you don't run into any trouble up there in California.

LINDA: I don't carry a gun, so that's okay. I'm in a pretty safe place, a very safe place. Very nice, high-end security job. I'm the person people see in the mornings when they come in all grumpy and wish they weren't there. They get to hear my voice first thing in the morning.

JOE: First thing in the morning. Now, does that make them *more* grumpy? Just kidding.

LINDA: No, it's true! They ask me, "How can you be so awake?"

JOE: Coffee.

LINDA: No, I don't drink coffee.

JOE: Oh, there you go.

LINDA: I'm just a morning person.

JOE: You're just a wake-up-and-go kind of person.

LINDA: Yeah, but don't ask me at nighttime.

JOE: Right. We're lucky to have you on here tonight.

LINDA: Thank you.

JOE: So, you were working with kids, running around all day, carrying them on your shoulders. When did you first start having health problems? What was your first major health issue?

LINDA: The major one was when I was diagnosed with high blood pressure.

JOE: You didn't believe them at first?

LINDA: Nope.

JOE: That's sometimes smart.

LINDA: Yeah, well, maybe not so smart *not* to believe them, but that was the beginning. My blood pressure was so high, but I was so young. I was only in my 20s.

JOE: So, in your 20s, you were diagnosed with high blood pressure?

LINDA: Yes, I was.

JOE: What did they do for you? What did they give you?

LINDA: Medication.

JOE: Drugs? Statins?

LINDA: No, not statins, just high blood pressure meds. They tried to bring it down. They even used nitroglycerin under my tongue to try to lower it.

JOE: Oh, wow.

LINDA: Yeah, I had a couple of trips to the hospital for it. My blood pressure was around 200 over something ridiculous.

JOE: So, you had to go to the hospital for that?

LINDA: Yep.

JOE: How long were you on the medication?

LINDA: I still am.

JOE: Oh, well, you shouldn't have told Dr. Reese that.

LINDA: Oh, he knows.

JOE: Well, that's got to be one of the goals, right?

LINDA: It is. My whole journey—my whole weight loss journey, everything—has been about getting off every med I was ever put on. And I'm off everything but that.

JOE: That's still a huge step.

LINDA: Yep.

JOE: What do they do if you go into the emergency room with a 200 blood pressure?

LINDA: They take you into a room, turn off the lights, make you lay there, and put nitroglycerin under your tongue for hours.

JOE: Basically, without saying it, they told you to *meditate*.

LINDA: Yep.

JOE: Ha! See, they know what works.

LINDA: They just don't call it that.

JOE: So, they basically told you to lay there, relax, and let the medicine do its job.

LINDA: Yeah, for three hours. Just lay there in the dark and do nothing. And I was mad as hell because I was supposed to be going out to dinner with Bill.

JOE: Right, so without officially saying it, they wanted you to just *chill out* and lower your stress levels.

LINDA: Exactly.

JOE: So, besides the high blood pressure, which could have led to other things, what other medical issues have you had?

LINDA: Well, what really started to draw me into looking for alternatives was my fertility issues. My first child was born, and then there was a nine-year gap before my second. In between that time, I didn't want my kids so far apart. But I couldn't carry a pregnancy. I lost eight babies in between my first and my second.

JOE: Oh, Linda, I'm so sorry to hear that.

LINDA: Everything happens for a reason, right? But it was a really difficult time. I ended up having major surgery, and then seven months later, I was pregnant. I had gone to a fertility specialist, and that was an interesting experience, to say the least. But then, I had two kids right in a row. My second child, and then 19 months later, my third. After that, I told them to undo what they did.

JOE: What did they do for you that finally allowed you to get pregnant?

LINDA: I had what they called adhesions blocking my tubes. My ovaries were stuck to the walls of my stomach. So, I had to have major surgery to remove all that, and once they cleared it up, I was able to get pregnant.

JOE: So, you've had surgeries.

LINDA: Oh yeah.

JOE: I know we've talked in this group before, but let's go over it again. So, you had high blood pressure, fertility issues, major surgery to fix your adhesions—what else?

LINDA: They gave me a knee replacement.

JOE: A knee replacement?!

LINDA: Yep, in my 30s.

JOE: Wow.

LINDA: And then both of my feet were reconstructed.

JOE: Wow. I remember we discussed that in one of the meetings.

LINDA: And that's when I got hooked on pain medication. They put me on oxycodone.

JOE: That stuff is no joke.

LINDA: No, it's not. And after that, I said *never again.* It was the hardest thing I ever had to come off of.

JOE: Were you able to get off it completely?

LINDA: Yes, but I'll tell you, I wanted to kill Bill so many times.

JOE: That's a movie, you know—*Kill Bill.*

LINDA: I know, but it was bad. I felt terrible for him because I was going through withdrawal, and he had to deal with me. But I got through it. And I promised myself I would never take it again, and I haven't.

JOE: Good for you.

LINDA: That's when I started looking for alternatives. A friend of mine told me about functional medicine.

JOE: Oh yeah, okay.

LINDA: That's when I stopped seeing traditional doctors.

JOE: Right, so you were looking for alternatives and started seeing a functional medicine doctor.

LINDA: Yeah. He did extensive blood work, which is when I found out I was in *kidney failure.*

JOE: Whoa. So, what did the medical monopoly do for your kidney failure?

LINDA: I *didn't* go to them.

JOE: *Good answer.*

LINDA: I stayed with my functional medicine doctor, and we started working on it. He put me on different herbs and supplements. But then, I found out about a program in San Diego called the *Optimal Health Institute.* I went there for three weeks, and I learned a whole new way of life. Meditation, yoga, proper nutrition—it changed everything for me.

JOE: So, you were already doing yoga, meditation, functional medicine *before* you even came into the reversal system?

LINDA: Yes.

JOE: But something was missing.

LINDA: Exactly. I was looking for relief from my back pain. Ever since I had a nine-pound baby, my back has *never* been the same. I had tried everything, but it still hurt. That's when my husband found Dr. Reese.

JOE: *Bill found him?*

LINDA: Yep. He was trying to help me because I was in pain all the time. And I knew my back wasn't the only issue—I just didn't realize how much else was wrong.

JOE: So, how's your back doing now?

LINDA: It still screams at me sometimes, but I scream back.

JOE: Ha! That's the spirit.

LINDA: But it *is* better. Some days, it has its moments, but I can tell it's improving.

JOE: That's progress.

LINDA: And you know what? Since joining this program, I've noticed some other unexpected benefits.

JOE: Like what?

LINDA: My hair.

JOE: Your hair?

LINDA: Yeah! My hairdresser asked me, *"Linda, what have you done to your hair?"*

JOE: *That's* always a good sign.

LINDA: I wasn't even trying to improve my hair, but it got thicker and healthier on its own.

JOE: Wow. That's a nice little bonus.

LINDA: And I had this lump on the inside of my gum that just *disappeared*.

JOE: Wait, what?

LINDA: Yep.

JOE: That's crazy.

LINDA: I know! I didn't even come in for that—I came in to fix my *back*.

JOE: And how are your kidneys now?

LINDA: *Normal.*

JOE: *Whoa.*

LINDA: I got blood work done recently, and every single marker has improved. My kidneys are functioning normally again.

JOE: And that happened *here*?

LINDA: Yep.

JOE: That's incredible.

LINDA: I mean, even my liver is better. I had fatty liver disease, but my numbers have improved.

JOE: So, before, you were a *mess*—but now?

LINDA: *Cleaning up the mess.*

JOE: That's right.

LINDA: I don't know where I'd be today if Bill hadn't given me Dr. Reese's book.

JOE: That's powerful.

LINDA: He was trying to help me because I was miserable. But now, I'm following the program, moving, exercising, and I walk three to four miles a day at work.

JOE: That's fantastic.

LINDA: I track my steps on my Apple Watch, and sometimes, at the end of the week, I realize I've walked a *marathon.*

JOE: Wow.

LINDA: And I see people online who are 100 years old, living like they're 50. I want that to be me.

JOE: And it *will* be.

LINDA: That's why I'm here. I listen to every meeting, always learning, always looking for what else I can do.

JOE: And that's why you're getting results.

LINDA: Yep.

JOE: Linda, this has been an *amazing* conversation. Thank you for sharing your story.

LINDA: Thank you.

JOE: And remember, folks—if Linda can do it, so can you. Keep showing up, keep doing the work, and we'll see you next week.

LINDA: Take care, everyone!

Arthritic Hip Pain Gone in 30 Days, GERD Gone, Neuropathy Pain Disappearing

DR. REESE: What about the hip pain and the pelvis?

DEBBIE: It's funny because before I started this program, it was just starting to get worse and worse. And if I was sitting for a long time and I'd go to get up to walk, I'd go, "oh gosh", you know, it would hurt. But since about day 30 or so, I haven't had any of it. And then I had a little bit of pelvic pain with it.

That's completely gone. I can't say how much better I feel with my stomach. I mean, I have been from GI specialist to GI specialist, my family doctor, and nobody has ever helped me all these years. And as soon as I started this program, everything changed for me. So I'm very, very thankful for that.

I just love you guys. It's so nice to be part of your community and I'm really enjoying it.

Selfie Video From Debbie

Hey, my name is Debbie. This is my Day 120 video. I started following Dr. Reese several months ago. I found him on social media, watched his videos, got his books, and read them all. And I thought, "Gee, this guy makes so much sense with everything he says." So, I decided to take the plunge, do something for myself for a change, and join the program.

It turns out I've had so many successes. I'm really happy that I joined—it's been well worth it. I lost 10 pounds just by eliminating the four poor foods, and that was really easy. Other than that, I've always had bad digestion all my life. I've been to specialist after specialist, and no one has really been able to help me—except to put me on medication. I never thought I would come off Nexium, but I have, and Dr. Reese's program helped me with that. I've now been off of it for months. My digestion has never been better.

Also, by about Day 30, the hip pain I was having—arthritis and groin pain from my hip—was making walking difficult. I knew that someday

I'd probably be in for a hip operation. But then, the pain disappeared, and now, going into my fifth month, it has never come back.

Probably the biggest reason I joined the program is that about three to four years ago, I was diagnosed with neuropathy in both of my feet. It was just horrible—24/7 pain. I was told by multiple doctors that there was nothing they could do for me. They tried to give me pain medication and just told me that I would have to learn to live with it. But by about Day 90 in Dr. Reese's program, I noticed my feet started feeling better.

One day, I was walking around and suddenly realized—I forgot about my neuropathy. Before, I always felt it. It was always there, always bothering me. But now, it has been getting nothing but better. I have maybe five or six really good days where my feet feel much better. I might have the odd bad day, but overall, it's just been improving.

I'm so thankful to Dr. Reese and his awesome coaches for this. I've been so lucky. They've been so good to me. The coaches have been incredibly attentive and have helped me so much—I really appreciate them.

I attended Dr. Reese's seminar back in May, and it was really nice to meet everyone in person. Everybody was wonderful. I met many of his other clients, and it gave me the chance to talk to them, hear about their experiences, and learn about their successes. They, too, are very happy with how things have turned out.

I can't imagine where I would be in my life right now without Dr. Reese. He has helped me so much, and I just want to say thank you for that. I look forward to continuing my journey with Peace Over Pain Clinic. As long as you guys are there, I plan on being there.

Thank you very much—it's been awesome. Thanks!

DIABETES GONE

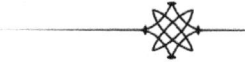

Ken: I did the 60-day blood sugar protocol diet. I finished that about less than a week ago. I can tell you, for a long time, I haven't seen any symptoms of type 2 diabetes. My blood sugar runs awesome. A lot of times during the day, it stays between 85 and 95. After eating, it might go up to 150, but it comes right back down within an hour.

I'm glad to say that we're done with that. I will be controlling it through my diet. I've also lost 30 of the 50 pounds you asked me to lose in just a little over two months. I've still got a little way to go, but I'm doing well.

DR. REESE: Well done. So, you jumped right into the blood sugar rescue, and it worked for you.

KEN: Yes, sir. And I guess that's what was causing me to lose weight too. Apparently, I was eating too much.

40 Symptoms Down to Just 10 Symptoms

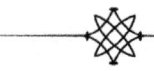

DR. REESE: Wow Bertha you went from 40 symptoms to 10 symptoms.

BERTHA: I'm feeling it. And my sleep is heavenly. Also, I ended up weighing myself this morning and I've lost 12 pounds

DR. REESE: Okay, your rashes are going away. No more nightmares and your bloating improved. And you said you had nightmares and they're gone now.

BERTHA: They're gone.

DR. REESE: Well, I think that's a testament to your blood sugar going from nine symptoms to two symptoms. Yeah. You know, that scale is just showing that you're getting out of the hole of a blood sugar issue. And the gut issue. That's pretty cool, you're on your way.

BERTHA: I am. I'm excited, I'm really excited. Thank you.

Knee Clicking Gone, Walking Pattern Restored

MITCHELLE: Before my knee would click whenever I go upstairs. And then whenever I travel, when I will be sitting in the car for like an hour, after an hour when I get up, my walking pattern is very bad. I couldn't even walk straight. And after doing PAT and after doing the nutrition, the vitamins and everything I don't have that anymore.

DR. REESE: It's gone, huh?

MITCHELLE: Yes.

DR. REESE: Just like that?

MITCHELLE: Yeah.

DR. REESE: And you said June.

MITCHELLE: June. So that's... The membership, I think I became a member, like when you started the membership. I'm trying to convince my husband, so now he's doing the PAT.

DR. REESE: You know those men are stubborn.

MITCHELLE: They are very, very stubborn.

Age Spots Gone, Panic Attacks Gone, Frozen Shoulder Gone, Migraines Gone, Low blood Sugar Gone

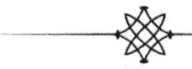

COACH SHAWN: Elise graduated her 120 last month. Postural therapy has been a game-changer. Age spots disappearing. Episodes have stopped where she was shaking, sweating, and having panic attacks and would almost pass out. Tunnel vision, and migraines are gone, and pressure in the head is all gone.

DR. REESE: Wow, Elise, that's pretty big.

ELISE: Thanks, Dr. Reese, you've changed the trajectory of my life. I've met so many amazing people and I've learned so much. I had a gnarly anterior pelvic tilt. Like I used to be a gymnast and I've always had it forever. I didn't even know that there was a term for it. I didn't, you know, and I don't have it anymore. Like Connor, whatever he's having me do is totally working. My frozen shoulder is gone too."

All Digestive Symptoms Massively Improving

DR. REESE: Priscilla, how better is your gut now, from where it was on day one to where it is right now?

PRISCILLA: My gut is much better, so much better. I wasn't able to eat meat for, I'm gonna say for at least two years or so. Since I've been in your program, I slowly implemented some meat into my diet. Burgers and chicken and fish, you know, and so it's much better. The digestive system is much better. I used to be so congested. I used to be so congested. It was just unbelievable. That has been a relief. Oh my goodness. Thank you so much for that.

COACH SHAWN: Remember in the beginning of the program with you you were struggling with like a lot of digestive issues Or just when you ate you had a lot of inflammation a lot of mucus and gastritis.

PRISCILLA: I feel good now. I mean like I mentioned before I'm able to eat now and keep food down and my digestive is just going well.

DR. REESE: And what about the pain?

PRISCILLA: No pain.

DR. REESE: It's gone?

PRISCILLA: It's gone. No tummy aches.

DR. REESE: Nothing in the joints?

PRISCILLA: No, my joints are lubricated. They feel great.

DR. REESE: Lubricated. All right. Yes, everything is going well, you know, doing what I'm supposed to do and just keep it moving. Okay.

PRISCILLA: Yes. Thank you so much. I'm thankful.

No Walker Needed, Sciatica is Gone

DR. REESE: So your sciatica is gone?

SUE: I really thought I was going to need a walker. In the very beginning I couldn't get out of bed. It was that bad. I'm very grateful. Absolutely. It's gone.

COACH SHAWN: Wow.

SUE: Thank you all. Thank you for being here.

COACH SHAWN: Thank you for having faith.

SUE: That I do.

DR. REESE: And you've been coming to the PAT classes on a regular basis?

SUE: Yes.

COACH SHAWN: I can attest to that. I see Sue in every posture class and it makes me happy. It just shows you like, you get out of the program what you put into it. So if you stay consistent, like Sue's a prime example, you stay consistent, you attend the classes, you ask questions. Look at that. Wow.

SUE: Are you on the 90 essential as well? Yes. Thank you so much.

DR. REESE: And so life is different now?

SUE: Yes. It really is. It's amazing because like I said before, I really thought I was gonna need a walker in the very beginning. I couldn't get out of bed. It was that bad.

Hernia Hump Gone

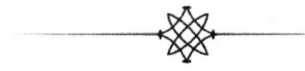

"I am on day 87 today. As far as updates are concerned, I have noticed that my energy levels are a lot higher. I'm less moody, especially with my kids. I feel like I'm more mellow and calm with them.

They don't stress me out so fast. As far as my physical appearance changes, I feel like my skin texture has improved a lot. My hump in my stomach has gone away. It's like a pre-hernia hump above my belly button. That's completely gone. So that's great. I hated that thing."

Period Pain Gone, Migraines Gone, Acne Gone, Constipation Gone

"So as you guys know I had you know a few problems with my body when I first started the program. Just to recap, I had problems with period pain and migraines, my hair was falling out I had a lot of acne and redness on my skin, my nails were really brittle, I had BM problems, and I'm really happy to say that a lot of the problems have gone away since I've been on this program.

You know, during this program I have not had a migraine or even a headache. My period pains are gone, and I don't have to take prescription pain pills anymore.

It feels really amazing to know that I'm not putting that in my body. My hair is thicker and I've had people comment or compliment on how shiny my hair is or how thick it is and how good it looks compared to before.

I've noticed my nails are a lot thicker. My skin is clear I've been told that I'm glowing now. I don't wear makeup on my skin and people are like, 'oh my God, your skin looks amazing', and it makes me feel good to know that other people are noticing it.

And I lost a total of 38 pounds on this program. I mean, in four months, I lost 38 pounds. Makes me feel amazing. I feel lighter, I feel happier."

TMJ Gone, Migraines Gone and Back Pain Gone

KAREN: When I first contacted you, I was actually kind of reflecting on conversations and my notes that have been taken throughout this process. That was one of the main reasons why I contacted you in the beginning back in December was TMJ. And honestly, I don't even know if I really had it. You always talk about the medical monopoly. I think the dental monopoly is just the same because I got in the chair and then they told me I had one problem and then I visited somebody else and they told me at another problem and then it escalated to where I had TMJ and then all of a sudden they fit me for this really expensive $4,000 appliance that I bought and then it changed my jaw and once I found you I was really excited because they were trying to convince me to do this protocol that was going to be $14,000.

DR. REESE: Whoa.

KAREN: And that wasn't even going to take care of all of my issues.

KAREN: I ended up ditching the appliance that I bought after wearing it for a few months, and then found you and started doing the protocols and my jaw went back into the place it was supposed to be, and my pain went away. I don't have my neck pain, my shoulder pain.

DR. REESE: So the migraines are gone?

KAREN: The migraines are gone. The upper back pain gone. The neck pain gone. The jaw pain gone too.

DR. REESE: In 120 days?

KAREN: Yeah, actually today's 122.

DR. REESE: There you go. That's awesome.

KAREN: And it went by so fast. So fast, I wasn't even counting the days. If I didn't look at my little chart to know what day it was, it didn't matter. Because I knew I was making progress.

KAREN: Like you said, don't get caught in your head.

KAREN: Before I used to, I felt like my brain was a pinball machine and all the thoughts were going all over the place and it was ringing and dinging and it could be during the daytime, nighttime when I woke up in the middle of the night and stuff like that. But my thoughts and my head, my brain is so much clearer now. And I did the session where you were talking about doing the meditation in the shower. So I did that yesterday and then I was like, "oh, I'm washing dishes".

KAREN: I'm gonna do it when I'm washing dishes, washing this plate, washing this fork, whatever. And I was so focused on the present that I forgot to go to my parent's house to help them in the morning.

KAREN: Then I had to call them, "I'm so sorry, I'm late. I'm gonna be an hour late." because I was caught up in the moment.

Interview with Karen

JOE: So when did you first start having difficulties with your health? What was your first *major* health incident?

KAREN: Probably in my late teens, early 20s—I dislocated my shoulder. I was playing racquetball with a friend, and apparently, just hitting the ball straight was enough for my shoulder to pop out of joint.

JOE: Oof.

KAREN: It went back in, but that was the start of my problems. Later, I started having other issues, but at the time, I just thought, *"Okay, loose joints, whatever."* I didn't realize it might be a posture issue.

JOE: Right, of course. The doctors never look that deep into it when you're young. If they had, maybe your shoulder wouldn't have kept popping out.

KAREN: Exactly. Over the years, it's happened at least ten times between both shoulders—probably more. I've lost count.

JOE: So now both shoulders pop out?

KAREN: Yeah. I used to just put them back in myself.

JOE: Wow.

KAREN: One time, I was swimming and hit the wall too hard—popped out. Another time, I was lifting weights—popped out. I was playing with my kids, sofa surfing—popped out.

JOE: Wait, *sofa surfing?*

KAREN: *Laughs* Yeah! We'd throw couch cushions on the floor, and I'd dive onto them. One time, my husband was out of town, and my kids had to help me put my shoulder back in.

JOE: That must have been a *fun* experience.

KAREN: *Laughs* Oh yeah.

JOE: So besides the shoulder, has anything else come up over the years that made you deal with the medical monopoly?

KAREN: Oh, for sure. I had a freak accident when I was younger—late teens. I was helping a friend with landscaping, and they accidentally cut through my leg.

JOE: *What?*

KAREN: Yeah. Severed three muscles right below my knee. It was bad.

JOE: Oh my God.

KAREN: I was lucky it didn't hit the bone or the main nerve. But ever since, I've had foot drop and nerve damage in that leg.

JOE: And did they give you physical therapy?

KAREN: No. They told me I *wouldn't be able to walk.*

JOE: *What?*

KAREN: Yep. But I told myself, *"No way. I'm going to run."* I refused to accept their prognosis.

JOE: *Bravo.*

KAREN: But it's affected my walking ever since. I fall sometimes because of that instability.

JOE: So, an injury at 18 threw your whole body off?

KAREN: Pretty much. And now, after all these years, I'm finally addressing it with postural therapy.

JOE: *That's* incredible.

KAREN: Yeah, it's amazing to see improvements in something I thought I'd just have to live with.

JOE: And that's why this program is so different. It actually *gets to the root cause.*

KAREN: Exactly.

JOE: So, what made you decide to become a coach?

KAREN: I saw how much this helped me, and I wanted to help others. When I first spoke to Tamara, I told her, *"I love what you do. Someday, I'd love to be a health coach."* And now I am.

JOE: That's fantastic.

KAREN: This program changed my life, and now I get to help others change theirs.

JOE: And that's why you're here. Karen, this has been an *amazing* conversation. Thank you for sharing your journey.

KAREN: Thank you!

JOE: And for everyone listening—*do the protocols, and you'll start to feel great.*

KAREN: Absolutely!

JOE: All right, Karen, thanks again.

KAREN: Talk to you soon. Bye-bye!

Ulcerative Colitis Gone!

"I was diagnosed in 2009 with ulcerative colitis. I was hospitalized several times. I was stuck inside a lot. The problem with ulcerative colitis is that you need to have a bathroom available almost all the time. So getting anywhere on time didn't happen.

I was at the disposal of having to go to the bathroom or having the pain to go to the bathroom. Road trips can't happen. I wasn't able to do a road trip. They said, well we could put you on another medication and another medication and another medication and you're going to have to learn how to deal with this. And this is a lifelong diagnosis. I was in tears. I really didn't want to go on more medication.

The first time I saw Kevin's book was when I was scrolling through Facebook.

I was intrigued. It taught you lots of basics. So I started doing that. I started to feel better. And to not be on medication anymore was a miracle, it seemed. But it also seemed too good to be true.

But I gave it a whirl. So a few weeks ago I had a colonoscopy and it came back as inactive colitis. I feel wonderful. My doctor told me not to change a thing. It completely changed my lifestyle. And it is the best I've felt in years."

Vocal Cord Regenerated

DR. REESE: So what was wrong with your vocal cord?

WOMAN: Well, I was scared into surgery. Whether or not it was necessary, I don't know, but he used all the horrible words, "you're going to have a stroke", and, "you're going to have a heart attack", and, "you're going to be in a wheelchair".

So I had the surgery and afterward I kind of sounded like a frog. He said, "oh, just give it a few days", or, "give it a few weeks", or, "give it a handful of months". So I finally went and had the thing put down my throat and they said, "oh yeah, your vocal cord is partially paralyzed, not working".

So I had already been hanging out on your Facebook page in the background for two years and I had already been off gluten for 10 years at that time, but I was like the French fry queen haha.

So I got rid of that (and it took a good year), but all of a sudden one day I went back for my final, like I'll go one more time and have them look at my vocal cord and it was working. There it is. No more frog sounding voice.

DR. REESE: So you got off the poor four foods and your vocal cord regenerated?

WOMAN: Yes.

DR. REESE: In one year?

WOMAN: Yep.

DR. REESE: Can't make this stuff up. You're not a paid actor?

WOMAN: No, I'm sure not.

DR. REESE: I didn't send you a thousand dollars?

WOMAN: No, but you can if you want.

DR. REESE: Very cool. That's really good to hear. You must have been very happy with that.

WOMAN: Yes, yes. I am very grateful.

DR. REESE: All that was happening was the free radical damage just happened to hit that area and then by getting off the poor four foods, it gave it a chance to regenerate.

Blood Sugar Down 154 Points

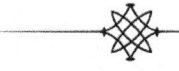

DR. REESE: What was your blood sugar before?

STEVE: Oh.. 270, 280, 260. After three times of doing cardio a day, I would still wind up with like 190 something at night, go to bed, then wake up in the morning with 270s, 280s, 260s, and struggle real hard. I actually went to a medical doctor today, and he checked me in his office. I was 126. I was really happy, he even tried to put me on ozempic today because I'm still obese, so I got to do your head to toe analysis. It's long overdue, man.

DR. REESE: Yeah, we got to get you in on the analysis so we can see what's going on and then we can fix it. We want to get that 126 blood sugar down to an 85.

STEVE: I agree. I'm just ashamed about how my body looks, but hey.

DR. REESE: No one needs to see it. We'll be the only ones.

STEVE: I hear ya.

Allergies Gone & Kidney Pain Gone

"Hi everyone, this is Lori and I am doing my 120 day video. Yay! Never thought this day would be here. I am just so happy.

I'm happy to report that my kidney pain is gone. I haven't had any kidney stones since starting the 120 day challenge.

I have no more allergies. I mean I may a tiny tiny bit but I don't take allergy medicine anymore. My allergy medicine I had to take every night. That was how I got to sleep because it makes you tired.

My immune system has been strong. When I was so overweight, I would get sick all the time, all the time.

Lab work came back phenomenal. My triglycerides went down over a hundred points. My liver enzymes came back excellent.

And my kids, my kids are my kids are so happy that I'm eating healthy. My little one loves my high-pitched noises.

Thank you Kevin."

Hand Pain Gone and Brain Fog Gone in 50 Days

DR. REESE: How are you feeling?

SONIA: Feeling good. Yeah, great progress as always. The hand pain, I can barely feel it. So another week of relief. I'm really, really pleased. Had a good chat with Coach Karen yesterday and can't thank her enough.

SONIA: She's such a great support. She really is. I was just saying to her how much the brain fog is gone, which I thought I'd gotten rid of, but it's just more layers and layers. The clarity that I've gotten is unbelievable. And then it brings on the confidence as well.

SONIA: So just the way it feels inside is amazing. I wasn't even expecting that part of it. There's so many bonuses that go along with this program that's just unreal. And I'm just 50 days in. That's the testament to it.

Chronic Stomach Pain Gone and Skin Blemishes Gone

"For two years I suffered from intestinal pains that would literally paralyze me. I would have to hold my breath, lay down flat on my stomach until it passed. So, I had black blemishes mostly on my armpits like on the bottom here. I probably never wore short sleeves because of it, I thought that I would never be able to. I also suffered from fatigue where every morning was five more minutes. I'm too tired to do this, too tired to do that. Since I did the program, the intestinal pains are gone, the blemishes on my skin are gone and I feel like every day is a great day and I'm ready to start it."

Pregnant Women Given 3 Months to Live...

"See the baby? He's in there, right? And can you see the tumor? This is the tumor. And this is the birth canal. And this is why they said that I couldn't get him out. The doctor told me that I needed to start to prepare. That I need to start to make final preparations. It is, um, really overwhelming. I guess there's probably a lot of words to say, but when the doctor tells you that you're pretty much done, and that I had like four more months until he was supposed to be born, that that was it.

And the only thing I could think to ask the doctor was, "am I going to even have enough time to see him? Am I going to bleed out so quickly that I won't even be able to ever see what he looks like?" But I went home and I did some research, went up and down my Facebook timeline and I saw Kevin on there talking about food and the way that we eat. So I called him up and I joined the program.

Two months later when I went back to the doctor to try to figure out how we were going to get the baby out, they couldn't locate the tumors.

On May 17th, I had my son with no complications, vaginally, and he's fine and we're fine. And I'm 100% under the belief that if I hadn't found Kevin, we would not be here."

Interview with Kim

COACH SHAWN: I'm here with Kim, and yeah, we're just gonna talk a little bit about her testimony with Dr. Reese and get to know a little bit more about her as well. So, really quickly, before we started, Kevin literally just told me that you were, like, from ten years ago.

KIM: Yeah, when he was K-Dub, he used to be on the radio.

COACH SHAWN: K-Dub?

KIM: Yeah, K-Dub is his radio name. He's popular, really popular—DJ on 93.7.

COACH SHAWN: How did you get involved with him?

KIM: He made an announcement on the radio that the radio station and the music, or whatever it was, wasn't in line with where he was going in his life. So that's interesting, right? So I started watching his social media—Facebook—and he started posting things about, like, humanitarian stuff. And then, like, it was very broad. And then he kind of narrowed down on food. Yeah, food and the effects of food and how that had a lot to do with companies' motivations and the way that people behave generally. And then he started to become more and more interested, so I watched him progress from K-Dub to Kevin Reese.

COACH SHAWN: To Dr. Kevin Reese. Yeah. Yeah, he has a good style with how he speaks in his videos. It's like drawing you in. So, um, what exactly—like, why did you go to him? What were you dealing with at the time?

KIM: I was pregnant. I think I was like 34, and I was pregnant. I got pregnant with my son, Michael. He wasn't Michael then, but I was pregnant. And at about five months pregnant, I went to the doctor. They do, like, your ultrasound. And when they did my ultrasound, they told me that I had—I wanna say—it was three tumors. One of them wasn't gonna be an issue, but two of them were. And I just wanna make this clear to you. One of them was the size of a grapefruit, and it was blocking the birth canal.

COACH SHAWN: Really?

KIM: Right from the back. Really. And then the other one was in the front, on the side. And so, apparently, if you cut a tumor, it causes hemorrhaging. So they weren't going to be able to cut them out, and I wasn't going to be able to push him out.

COACH SHAWN: Did you know that they were there, or did you just...

KIM: The tumors? No, not at all. Like that, because you can't feel them.

COACH SHAWN: Really?

KIM: No, I didn't know they were there. I felt fine. I felt absolutely fine. Everything was fine all the way up until they were doing the ultrasound because that stuff just kind of looks like static.

COACH SHAWN: Yeah.

KIM: You know? Yeah. And so the doctor—he said, "Oh boy, you have two large tumors that are gonna block your birth canal, and it's gonna make delivery of this baby impossible. And you need to get your affairs in order."

COACH SHAWN: Yeah. What was going through your head when that happened?

KIM: Nothing.

COACH SHAWN: Well, you were just, like, in shock?

KIM: Yeah, you just kind of go blank. Alright, that's it.

COACH SHAWN: What do they call that—radio silence?

KIM: Yeah. What did he just say? I was gonna die? Like, what does that mean? Yeah, get my affairs in order—no, I don't even have any affairs. Like, I'm 34, but I'm not old enough to have affairs.

COACH SHAWN: Wait, so this was just an appointment to check on the child?

KIM: Oh my gosh. Yeah, I'm going in, I'm gonna see him, right? Because every mom—you want to hear the heartbeat. You know, this is, like, a pretty exciting thing. You know that mothers look forward to this. You go and you get the ultrasound, you hear the heartbeat, you see the little toes, and they say, *Look, he's got five toes!* And, you know, they tell you the sex if you want to know. But not me. He said I was going to die. And, well, he said—this is a Mercy hospital, a religious hospital. He used a different word. But basically, they save the baby and not the mother.

COACH SHAWN: Okay...

KIM: So I don't know what bleeding out means. I mean, does that happen quickly? Like, how fast? Am I going to see him?

COACH SHAWN: Yeah.

KIM: You know what I mean? And so I'm thinking, *Oh my God, okay, so this is going to go down. Am I going to have the thing on my face or whatever? Am I going to, like, bleed out, lose consciousness? Am I going to see him first? Is that ever, you know, what's going to happen here?* So, and the doctor—he just got up and left. It was like he was really angry about it.

COACH SHAWN: Angry?

KIM: Yeah. Because I think that at 34, I was gonna give birth to him at 35, but at 34, they were supposed to take some precautions. And so, probably, they would have recommended that I get an abortion if they had given me an ultrasound sooner.

COACH SHAWN: Yeah.

KIM: But at that point, it was too late to give me an abortion or anything. They couldn't do anything. I couldn't get him out without dying. *Die, die, die.* So I drive home, right? And I don't know—it kind of puts life into a different perspective, right? So now what, right? So now I'm bringing this baby into the world, and they're not gonna have a mom. And they're not gonna have a mom—like, immediately.

COACH SHAWN: Yeah, that would—yeah.

KIM: Yeah. They're gonna go to the room where they keep all the babies, and this particular baby is not gonna have a mom.

COACH SHAWN: Right.

KIM: So I started doing research on these tumors—like, what are they?

COACH SHAWN: You went straight to work?

KIM: Yeah. *Why can't they get rid of them?* I don't want him to not have a mom. That's like the worst thing in the world. I love my son—even now—but when I was pregnant with him, I was so happy. *Oh my God. Oh my God. I was so happy I was pregnant. It was like the best pregnancy ever. This was the nicest little boy—the whole time I was pregnant. I just was so happy. I was so—*

COACH SHAWN: Did you have, like, dreams of him?

KIM: Yeah. I just felt like... Moms know their children so well. You know? There's no separation when you're pregnant. He kind of mellowed me out. Like, I was nervous to do the interview today, but if I was pregnant with my son, I wouldn't have been. I mean, he just made things—like, Lionel Richie has a song, I think it's called *Easy*. You know, *That's why I'm easy, easy like Sunday morning.* He had that vibe.

COACH SHAWN: Really?

KIM: So, love, right? I don't want him to not have a mom. So what can I do? How am I gonna either find him a mom or figure out—like, I need this kid to have a mom. And so, I started researching like, *Well, what are these tumors?* Because the doctor didn't really explain anything to me. He just said, *You know, you're gonna die.*

COACH SHAWN: Yeah, that's crazy.

KIM: He didn't say that exactly. He just said, *Get your affairs in order.* But nobody came in after to explain to me what that actually meant. So, I started searching online. And these tumors—I believe—are formed from estrogen when you're pregnant. And as the baby grows, the tumors grow. So, the more pregnant I became, the bigger they were gonna get, right?

COACH SHAWN: So there was no way around it?

KIM: Because if they cut me from the back—right—my kidneys and my liver are back there. They can't do that, right? And if they cut me from the front, I bleed to death, and I can't push him out. So, they weren't going to take the risk of doing the surgery because I just—I wasn't going to make it. My body was going to continue to feed the tumor.

COACH SHAWN: Yeah.

KIM: If they removed it, there was some issue. So these tumors—they're fed by estrogen, bad food, stress, you know, and just—everything amounted to the food I was eating and my body's ability to process toxins and waste in the way it needed to. Stress. Basically, not taking care of myself, not paying attention. Not drinking water. *Water—deep water, lemon water, things like that. Very basic stuff. Leafy greens.* And so, I remembered K-Dub—Kevin Reese—had been talking about this stuff. So I went to his page. He had a recipe on there. I looked it up, and I made it. I started following his page every day—like, I was watching him. He was doing live videos. I was on them, watching his stuff. I went out and got the ingredients. And when I first tasted it, I was like, *Oh, this stuff is terrible.*

COACH SHAWN: Yeah?

KIM: Yeah. But I drank it. And I felt better.

COACH SHAWN: Really?

KIM: Yeah, because you can feel it. It's tingly—you know what I mean? You feel it. And so, it was good. It wasn't, you know—it wasn't terrible. A week goes by, and he had a group you could join where they supported you as well. Because part of what I was going through was stress, too. And what's more stressful than *I'm gonna die?* I think I had, like, three months.

COACH SHAWN: Three months left?

KIM: Yeah. So, I joined the support group. And he gave me more tips on how to eliminate. But at this time, I didn't tell him, like, *Oh, I'm* *dying.* Because that sounds so—I don't know—it just sounds so sad. I didn't want to, like, you know—I don't know. I didn't talk to him about it. But I was doing what he said to do. He had a morning routine, a lunch routine, a dinner routine. Like, *This is how you take care of yourself.* And every day, it was more and more of what you do and how you take care of yourself.

COACH SHAWN: Wow.

KIM: So, I switched over to a different hospital—Hartford Hospital. Because the previous hospital—it was, like, a religious hospital, whatever type of hospital it is where they don't save the mom. But Hartford Hospital does everything they can to save both people. It's a teaching hospital. So, I transferred over there. And when they did the ultrasound—there were no tumors.

COACH SHAWN: Wow.

KIM: Yeah. So, this is probably about a month, a month and a half later—no tumors. Right. So, they sit me on the table, and they do the regular—you know, they put the lube on me, and then they're doing the thing. And she's like, *I don't see anything.* And so, she starts jamming me. And she's jamming hard. And, you know, it really shouldn't be that hard because at this point, I'm, like, six and a half or seven months or something.

COACH SHAWN: Yeah.

KIM: She's really digging. I remember her specifically digging into this side.

COACH SHAWN: She was looking for it?

KIM: Yeah. Nothing. They even had me turn to my side to see, you know, what they could see. Then she's like, *Alright, we're going to try another way.* So, they get this thing, and it's like—*You know, we're going to try it from the inside.*

COACH SHAWN: Oh wow.

KIM: So now, I'm up in the stirrups, right? And they're trying it from the inside—jamming it, jamming that thing. I was like—you know—I'm telling her, *That hurts!* She's like, *You gotta relax.* And I'm like, *I'm relaxed! That hurts!* She's like, *I just really want to make sure we find it because I don't see what the ultrasound said. The records that they sent aren't matching what I'm seeing.*

So, she leaves the room. She seems all upset and confused. It's a conundrum now, right? Like, *What is this?* She goes out, gets somebody else, and now they're jamming me too. She's got a second opinion. She's got another person jamming me—nothing.

COACH SHAWN: Wow.

KIM: So, I get dressed, make another appointment, and I go home. They don't tell me anything conclusive. Nothing. Nothing. I go back to the next appointment, and now they got the doctor—like, the big doctor or whatever. And he does the thing—you know, everything that she did—but he was a lot more gentle. And he was like, *There are no tumors here.*

COACH SHAWN: Wow.

KIM: Yeah. There were no tumors. So now, I'm at the point where they start to schedule the delivery. *If you don't have the baby by this time, then we're going to induce your labor,* or whatever.

COACH SHAWN: So, two months?

KIM: Yeah. It took, like, no time at all. No tumors. Tumors gone. They totally disappeared. I wasn't in a high-risk pregnancy anymore—nothing. And I left out of the doctor's office that day, and I was having a baby. I was having a baby boy. I was having a baby in, like, a month and a half. And now, you know—the whole world is different.

COACH SHAWN: What's the baby's name?

KIM: Michael.

COACH SHAWN: Michael.

KIM: Yeah.

COACH SHAWN: That's a miracle baby.

KIM: Yeah.

COACH SHAWN: How old is he now?

KIM: Michael is 10. Michael is actually being scouted by the middle schools in our area for, like, high-achieving or exceptional students.

COACH SHAWN: Wow.

KIM: Yeah, a very smart kid. Michael took the SATs—I think the fourth-grade SATs—and he passed. I guess his score was high enough to get into college.

COACH SHAWN: Wow, really?

KIM: Yeah. So now, he's going to go to a special school. They just recently scouted him for it. I'm immensely grateful. I'll never be able to pay Kevin back. I want to so badly give him something for what he gave me. But he doesn't even understand.

COACH SHAWN: Yeah.

KIM: He's just like, *It's yours.* Everything is so easygoing with him. Like, *Yeah, you just gotta do this, this, and that, and things just flow.*

COACH SHAWN: Yeah.

KIM: He always says that. *It just flows.* But for me? My son almost didn't have a mom. For me, that's the end of the world. For him, it's just like, *It's the flow.* But for me, you know—you stopped the end of the world. It's a big deal.

COACH SHAWN: It's a big deal. I mean, I believe he saved my life too. So, like, I think our stories—at the end of the day—I believe your story is one of the most powerful I've ever heard.

KIM: Wow.

COACH SHAWN: It was actually one of the stories that got me on board. Your story is helping save people—so many lives. Even the people who aren't necessarily dying, but who are, like—I wasn't dying per se, but I was in so much pain, and I didn't know what route to take. And I'm sure you know—when you're researching, you see all these conflicting facts and opinions. And the doctors are on you about everything, and they're getting mad at you. And these are the people that you're supposed to look up to, you know? But—no compassion at all. Then you see Kevin, and it's like a whole different perspective on health and life.

KIM: Right.

COACH SHAWN: So, I just think that what you're doing here—thank you for coming back and sharing this.

KIM: Oh my God. I wish I could do more. Yeah. Like, yeah, I really—like, I didn't want to be in front of the camera and all of that. But I'm just like, *I have to do something.* And so—he has a TikTok now, right? So, I follow him on TikTok. And I would see people commenting things like, *Oh, she's making it up.*

I wouldn't. I just wouldn't. I'm not that type of person. I wouldn't waste my time doing that. I'm just a grateful person. And, you know, I do have a great relationship with my son. Because I had him at the age that I did, it allowed me to be the mother I always wanted to be. I was able to be somebody that I never even imagined I could be. And just like that—you know—the doctor comes in the room and tells me, *You need to get your affairs in order.*

All of my dreams—you know what I mean? There were no opportunities. Because that's the end of opportunities. And then—

thank God. No, I'm right—thank God. Because, absolutely, for him— I guess, for him, it's like, *Well, this is my purpose.* But thank God that your purpose aligned with mine. Because had they not... You know?

COACH SHAWN: Yeah.

KIM: Here's the thing, right? I love my son so much that if I hadn't been here to have him—who would have loved him like me? Nobody can love a son or a child like their mother. He's so beautiful, too. It's just— the relationship that we have, it wouldn't have been possible. I really, really wanted to be his mom. And Kevin—he gave that back to me.

COACH SHAWN: You want some tissues?

KIM: No. Thank you. I developed so much into a woman because of being able to be a mom. And he just gave me the opportunity back. And it almost wasn't there. You don't even know—it almost didn't happen. It just almost didn't happen. That's all. It just wouldn't have happened. And I would have been, like—how many other people?

COACH SHAWN: Yeah.

KIM: How many other people lay on that table, and they say, *You know, that's it, you're done?* Or how many women lay down without them even finding it? You know? During the ultrasound? And they just hemorrhage out unnecessarily. Anything could have happened. But something different happened for me. And because of that—there are so many opportunities. You know what I mean? And so now, my son is in the gifted and talented program, and I'm gonna be able to see him live his dreams. I love every minute of it. All because of some nasty shakes. It's crazy.

COACH SHAWN: It wasn't even just the nasty shakes, though.

KIM: It was him. Like—I believed him.

COACH SHAWN: Yeah.

KIM: Yeah, I believed him. Because if I didn't believe him, I would have just kept scrolling. I don't know. It's one of those things. I think I did it because I took that risk, but—

COACH SHAWN: Desperation?

KIM: You mean, like, I had the willingness of the desperate? Yeah.

COACH SHAWN: Like, you were trying to save you and your son's life. To me, that's not even desperation. Doctors weren't giving you the answer that you needed, so you had to search for it. And just like you were saying—what if you hadn't searched for it? What if you had just accepted it?

KIM: Right. Back then, I was one of—well, I don't even know how many people live in America. But I was one of those people who believed— what the doctor says is right. The doctor's word is absolute. And all the way until my back was against the wall, I still believed that. Then I was like—I have to find hope. There's got to be a way. Yeah. There's got to be a way.

COACH SHAWN: Why does it have to take that much?

KIM: Money, I guess.

COACH SHAWN: Yeah, I mean—so much. Does your son—does he know the story?

KIM: Yeah. Well, no. He got older, and then—I'd say, you know, we'd be out hiking or something, and I'd say, *This almost didn't happen.* You know? I'm so grateful. And I want him to know, too. I'm extremely grateful. I'm grateful for him. I love him so much. I'm excited by him. He's funny. He's witty. He's got this big curly hair. Right now, he's really into his iPad. And, you know, he's kind of growing into his own thing. We're not as close as we used to be, but—it's all healthy. And I'm able to watch him and see him.

COACH SHAWN: Well, you know—it comes back around. I know that when me and my mom were, like, super, super, super close, then the teenage years came. But once everything—this is just reassurance for you. You probably already know.

KIM: He'll come back. He'll come back. You know, but I'm still—I don't know. Just being able to have him and watch him, and be a part of the whole thing, and just, you know—hear his jokes. I don't know. He's dope. He talks about philosophy, society, and the community. His thoughts—he says things from perspectives that are fresh. These are fresh new perspectives. From a young person. He really is an amazing, amazing human being. He really is. I really like him. I love him, but I like him, too. You know what I mean? Because he's very interesting. Very interesting. He's very smart. His ideas are new and fresh and free.

COACH SHAWN: That's beautiful.

KIM: He's easy. Like Sunday morning.

COACH SHAWN: I'm going to have that song stuck in my head now.

KIM: Yeah. Peaceful. He's an extremely peaceful kid. I don't know. It's been a great experience. I'm glad. I don't think too much about what could have happened. Because—I'm alive. I don't have any understanding of what death would have been. You know? I'm just here. A mom. And I'm here to help guide him to where he needs to be.

COACH SHAWN: And he's gonna be really good for the community, too.

KIM: You know, I was able to help him out.

COACH SHAWN: Do you think that being confronted with death itself made you more grateful for life?

KIM: It does make me grateful for experiences that I have with people. Yeah. So, you want to have more experiences, right? And I want to be healthy. But what I did find out is that food is extremely addictive. And those types of long-term changes—they take dedication. You actually have to change your life. You know what I mean? And so, I'm grateful for life. But with that—with the information that he gave me... Like, we talked about parasites. Oh, I was one of the worst. But because of that, I—so now I have anemia. Well, I don't now, right? I don't have anemia now. When they told me that I did, I went and did something like a parasite cleanse. And so now, they're like—*Well, we don't know why your numbers changed.* I would have never looked if it wasn't for Kevin. You know what I mean? I would have never even been like—*Maybe you don't know what you're talking about. Maybe you're not doing all the right tests that you should be doing.* So I did this, this, and that. Which, basically, always goes back to a cleanse. A cleanse. Living right. Sleeping well. Drinking enough water. Things start to pan out.

COACH SHAWN: That's not taught at all. You have to dig for it. It's not even about finding it.

KIM: Yeah. I've noticed that it's weird. Or—I say weird, but it's just like... If you eat well and take care of your body, and that's important to you—it looks a lot different than what everybody else is eating and doing.

COACH SHAWN: Yeah.

KIM: Man, it's tough. But there really isn't any catch. I did it, you know? He made these recommendations. I took the recommendations. And now—I'm alive. There's no catch. There's no conspiracy. It's not rocket science. It's extremely simple.

COACH SHAWN: What does he say? Oh, yeah—he says, *It's so easy, it's hard.*

COACH SHAWN: Like, people are like, *That's it? That's all I have to do?* And they don't believe it.

KIM: Yeah.

COACH SHAWN: They're like, *No, this is fake.* And it's like, *There's only so much we can do.* He says it like that, but it will change you.

KIM: Yeah. Just like when he was on the radio station, and he was like, *This is not really in line with who I see myself becoming.* And it just—it's like that. That's how it is. When you start to respect yourself.

COACH SHAWN: That's deep.

KIM: It's a struggle. Yeah, I struggle with it. It's difficult—like, me and chocolate. And I know better. So it's like—I struggle with even things as simple as water.

COACH SHAWN: Yeah.

KIM: Or, for me, it just all boils down to self-respect. Now that there's no imminent danger—like, *if I don't do this, I'm going to die*—then it comes down to, *Well, what quality of life do I want?* How vibrant do I want to be? How upright do I want to stand? How much memory do I want to be able to recall? Because if I'm lethargic, and anemic, and not sleeping well, and all dehydrated—what kind of quality of life is that?

COACH SHAWN: And even later down the line, you'd just be sitting in bed all day. Like, one of those doctors that conflict with Kevin—they hate Kevin. One of them said something like, *People are living longer than ever before.* And I'm like—Are they really living? Is sitting in your bed, in your own urine, sometimes on meds—

KIM: Yeah.

COACH SHAWN: On meds. That's living? I mean, I want to live my life like that until I'm, what—80? And then that's living to them?

KIM: The point is working.

COACH SHAWN: Oh, yeah. They're bringing up the room.

KIM: I mean, my thought is—Kevin is a healer, right? But here's the thing: doctors treat sickness. So, you have to stay sick for them to have business, right? But Kevin—he works in health and healing. And healing is lifelong. You'll always be healing. And it's infectious. I go around to other people, and I'm like, *Oh, you know—* And they see me, and they're listening to what I'm saying, and they're like, *Oh, that's different.* And it plants little seeds in their minds. Which kind of takes business away from over here.

COACH SHAWN: Yeah, they don't like that.

KIM: They can't do it. And I think a lot of it has to do with addiction, as well. They put stuff in the food to keep you eating that stuff. And then the doctors treat you. They don't cure you—they treat you. So they can have you live as long as possible while treating you for as long as possible.

COACH SHAWN: Exactly.

KIM: So, every time doctors say something, you know—

COACH SHAWN: It's the opposite way. I remember one time—my grandpa had colon cancer. And they gave him a number of days. He stayed in the hospital, and I remember going down to the cafeteria— And there was a McDonald's in the hospital.

KIM: Wow.

COACH SHAWN: We ate it. I mean, this was at a time when I didn't know any better. But looking back on that, I'm like—*That doesn't make sense.* We're supposed to be eating healthy. You have all these health recommendations. But all these nurses, all these doctors, as well as the patients, are eating McDonald's?

KIM: Yeah. The last time I ate McDonald's, I think I was in North Carolina. I was starving. Pulled over on the side of the road. And there was no little mom-and-pop place, like where they sauté the onions and peppers. So, we get McDonald's. And I bite the burger. I'm so hungry. But I'm like—*It tastes weird.* I don't know what it is. And then I'm just like, *Okay, gulp it down. Whatever. Just drink it. Eat it.* I got it with water, too—just, *Okay*. And then I took another bite. And I'm like, *This is not what they're saying it is.* And then—even if it was beef—how am I ever gonna get this back out? I actually went into the bathroom and threw it up.

COACH SHAWN: Wow.

KIM: Yeah, I would rather be stuck. Because—what am I going to do with that? What's that going to do to me? It's not really worth it. I don't know what I'm getting into here. This is more than I'm bargaining for. Something's not right with this. The last time I had McDonald's, I actually went into the bathroom—inside the restaurant—and threw it up.

COACH SHAWN: As I said—that's where it belongs, to me.

KIM: Yeah.

COACH SHAWN: That's gross.

KIM: Insane. Even their fries—what the hell is in those?

COACH SHAWN: Yeah, they did a study. Somebody put seven different bags of fries from various restaurants in separate containers. And they let them sit for, like, a month. Every one of them molded—except McDonald's fries. And then people were still arguing it. They were like, *Oh, well, what did you do to it?* Or they just made up any excuse they could think of—other than, *Wow. What is in my food?*

KIM: If the air can't break it down...

COACH SHAWN: Yeah!

KIM: Then why can I break it down?

COACH SHAWN: Exactly.

KIM: But, you know—it tastes good. And it makes you feel better. At least, immediately. It makes you feel better. Leaves are not exciting.

COACH SHAWN: No.

KIM: Leaves are not exciting. That was my diet most of the time, growing up. All I ate was McDonald's. Anything fast food. I hated salads. I hated vegetables. And that's why I ended up how I did. But nobody was telling me that I needed to stop, necessarily.

COACH SHAWN: Yeah.

KIM: I mean—why would they? Everybody's doing it. If we're all doing it, then why... You must be sick for some other reason. Because we're all displaying sick behavior.

COACH SHAWN: Yeah. And now—it's a joke. Even the "itis," or something like that. Everybody just laughs about it. Or they're like, *Oh, I've got indigestion.* And it's like—*That's your body literally telling you something is wrong.*

KIM: Yeah.

COACH SHAWN: It's tough. Well, it's been a pleasure speaking with you.

KIM: Yeah, thank you. Go save some lives, guys.

Scoliosis Reversing in 70-Year-Old Woman!

DR. REESE: Last week I talked with Suzy and Suzy, you kind of made it sound like you didn't know if things were going well, but I looked at your photos and you're straight.

SUZY: Yeah, I'm glad you did that because it gave me a lift. I mean, I was shocked. I really was because it was clear to me that something had gotten better. I was straighter. Way straighter.

Plantar Fasciitis Gone and Knee Pain Gone

DR. REESE: So your knee pain is gone?

DENISE: Knee pain is gone.

DR. REESE: How long were you suffering from knee pain?

DENISE: The knee pain has been on and off. I was told that it was arthritic and they were talking about doing surgery. That was back in 2012. everything that I've been doing in the 120 has helped so that I don't feel it. I don't feel the knee pain anymore. And of course not aggravating it by wearing heels and I've been doing what you said, walking around the house barefoot.

I thought that my plantar fasciitis would come back, but it didn't. I've been just fine.

DR. REESE: So not only is your knee pain gone, but your plantar fasciitis is gone.

DENISE: Well, that was gone, but I thought it was because of the orthopedic devices that I was using in my shoes and orthopedic-type shoes. But since I dismissed them and I started walking without those devices, I thought that I was going to aggravate that, but I just took the step and kept on walking around in the house, in this house, and in the other house back in Indiana, and it has not come back, period.

DR. REESE: Okay. We'll chalk that up to a big victory then.

DENISE: Well, it's a victory for me. I don't know how you all look at it, but it's a victory for me.

DR. REESE: Yeah, no, it's a victory for us, too. And getting your husband on board is probably the biggest one of all, because men are stubborn.

DENISE: You don't have to tell me that!

"I just wanted to underscore that the process is improving. Everything is improving. And I don't plan on quitting because once I start something, I continue. So for anybody, any of the members that have any doubts, don't doubt it. Just take in everything because it can help you. And all the education is there. It's in the membership. So all you have to do is join. Get your head to toe analysis and then you proceed from there. It's really not hard. Dr. Reese and the team has made it easy. So thank you Dr. Reese for everything. God bless you. I continue to pray for you all and keep safe and blessings for the new year for you and everybody."

- Denise J.

Hypertension, Cysts, Stomach Pain, Migraines Gone

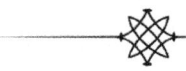

"So seven years ago, my doctor diagnosed me with high blood pressure and I was told it was hereditary and put on medication. Throughout that entire seven years, I had major anxiety over it. I felt like I was too young to have this and at any point, it was going to take me out. I felt like it was going to eventually kill me. I also had stomach pain, migraines, and lumps in my thigh. The doctors had no idea what the lumps were.

They threw a couple of different things out at me that were not the problem at all. So I was reluctant to join Dr. Reese because my doctor told me it was hereditary. I've tried a few things before that never worked. I finally decided to give it a try and within a couple of months, my doctor lowered my medication and two weeks later I was completely off.

Now I feel great. No more high blood pressure after seven years, no more medication, my body is not in pain anymore, my lumps are gone, swelling is gone." - Amber

Conquering Depression, Arthritis, and Weight Loss: Dr. Reese's 120-Day Challenge Transformed My Life

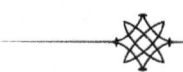

"Day 120 of the 120-day challenge, and right off the bat, I gotta say this—I feel healthy as f***. I've battled depression for over 20 years now, and I don't have any depression anymore. As far as... Well, the other thing would be my rheumatoid arthritis. All I can say is that it's one hundred percent manageable without any medicines—no medicines, no prescription medicines.

My beard? I would never grow it out before because it would have patches. That doesn't happen anymore. I've gotta go back for a lineup, but now I can grow it out. I can grow my beard!

Weight loss? I lost 25 pounds total during the 120-day challenge—25 pounds. I even ran out of notches on my belt! I had a size 38 belt, and I couldn't tighten it anymore because there were no more notches. So, I know it's time for me to buy new jeans, new clothes."

Arthritis Gone in 30 Days

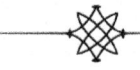

DR. REESE: 60 days in you have no more neck pain, huh?

LEEANN: Oh my gosh, I can't believe it. Especially on a day like today, we have a snowstorm going on right now and the humidity and the barometric pressure and everything, my neck would be so hot and so painful right now. And it's nothing.

DR. REESE: So how does that feel? Good?

LEEANN: It feels great. I'm amazed. I just can't, I'm like wow my neck isn't bothering me and it hasn't for a good month I think probably. It's been a while. Well my knees too but yeah my neck even when I went to get an adjustment she adjusted it a lot easier than normal.

DR. REESE: Very good.

Interview with Leeann.

COACH SHAWN: What exactly attracted you to the clinic and Dr. Reese?

LEEANN: So I came across him on social media, and pretty much everything he was talking about—I did watch a lot of his videos—and it's like, yes, yes, it's right. You know, I just believed pretty much everything he was saying. And the issues that I was having, it's like, geez, I wonder if that can be reversed as well, as with the way he was talking about everything. And he did mention the issues that I was having. So going forward and, you know, aging, I knew it was going to get worse if I didn't do anything. So I wanted to do something, but I didn't want to go to the doctors because they were just gonna give me injections and pills or whatever.

LEEANN: Exactly, so I definitely wanted to avoid that, but I knew I had to do something.

COACH SHAWN: I wanted to ask you, what were some of the symptoms that you had, if you don't mind?

LEEANN: Oh, no, no. I had chronic joint pain. Really. And I had a lot of arthritis in my neck and my lower back from an injury many, many years ago. I had ruptured discs in my neck and lower back. And as I got older, they didn't bother me that much when I was younger. This happened when I was probably in my 20s, so a long time ago. And so it didn't really bother me as I was aging until I started getting into my 50s and 60s, and then it was like, oh boy.

LEEANN: I started going to a chiropractor about eight or nine years ago, and he's like, oh yeah, you've got arthritis in your neck and your back, and you need to see me two times a month. And I did. I went to him twice a month for eight years.

COACH SHAWN: Wow.

LEEANN: It managed it maybe a little bit, but it would always come back—and always with a vengeance, too. I mean, just to the point where I couldn't turn my neck. It wasn't good. I also had shoulder pain, hip pain, knee pain. Well, like I told Levi when I first talked to him, I was in pain from head to toe.

COACH SHAWN: Oh my gosh.

LEEANN: So knees, ankles, and you know, I'm thinking, geez, if I don't do anything, I'm going to end up with surgeries and this and that.

COACH SHAWN: And so with all that, how do you feel now?

LEEANN: Once getting on the program, after 30 days, it reduced a lot. After 60 days, it was pretty much gone. I mean, I'm still amazed that my neck and my lower back do not bother me. And the chiropractor never did anything for eight years that I saw him multiple times a month. But yeah, after 60 days, pretty much gone. And I noticed it mostly in the beginning from my neck and my lower back. The exercises, postural therapy, definitely helped with that.

LEEANN: Especially my lower back, yeah. And the neck, I'm sure, too—everything. But yeah, pretty much everything. By day 60, it was pretty much gone.

COACH SHAWN: Did your progress pictures shock you every time?

LEEANN: They did, yeah. Just some exercises on the ground—it doesn't make sense, but it works, you know. And it feels so good too.

COACH SHAWN: Yeah.

LEEANN: Yes, very relaxing.

COACH SHAWN: Yeah, static back.

LEEANN: Oh my gosh, that's the go-to. I tell everybody, everybody needs a bit of static back.

COACH SHAWN: But with that being said, what was the most challenging part of being on the program, in your opinion?

LEEANN: Well, the gluten wasn't, because I was already gluten-free for eight years.

COACH SHAWN: So that was easy for you.

LEEANN: Yeah, that was like, okay, that's no big deal. The oils maybe were a little bit of a change. The fake and fried foods—not so much. Yeah, that was easy. But probably the oils were the hardest.

LEEANN: And then just getting into a routine in the beginning. So it's great to have the coach there for you. That's a definite plus. Yeah, I don't think I could have done it without the coaching. Not at all. There's just so much, and you know, they're there with you.

LEEANN: And if you have any questions, they help you in the beginning, setting everything up. Yeah. It's just overwhelming. So you need that support, definitely.

COACH SHAWN: Yeah, you trying to do that on your own?

LEEANN: No, I couldn't.

COACH SHAWN: Supplements, posture?

LEEANN: No.

COACH SHAWN: No?

LEEANN: No.

COACH SHAWN: How do you handle the peer pressure part of cutting the poor four foods?

LEEANN: Not bad with family dinners because I was eating pretty healthy anyway, other than the oil. And sugar—I was a big sugar person, so I had to cut a lot of that out. So family dinners weren't an issue. Everyone knows that I've been gluten-free, and I cook pretty much real food anyway—vegetables and meat. I keep it simple. The one thing was going out to dinner with friends, which I enjoy doing and still do. Probably not as much now, but yeah, that's a struggle sometimes.

LEEANN: Because you know, food and friends—it's just kind of like, you know, you get together, and so yeah, it's like a social thing.

COACH SHAWN: Definitely social.

LEEANN: Yeah, definitely.

COACH SHAWN: Have any of your friends or family members seen your progress and been led to look into the clinic at all?

LEEANN: They have seen the progress, yes—the weight loss and the fact that I don't have the pain anymore that I had. I mean, not too many people knew because I really didn't talk about it. It's just not me. So my son, you know, my immediate family, my mother.

COACH SHAWN: So getting the bad out of the way, what did you enjoy most about the program?

LEEANN: The fact that I was pain-free, pretty much.

COACH SHAWN: That's a great motivator.

LEEANN: Definitely.

COACH SHAWN: I mean, I was in so much pain.

LEEANN: And I knew it was going to get worse if I didn't do something. And I knew the doctors couldn't do anything. I just knew it. Yeah. So getting out of pain was the best motivator for me.

COACH SHAWN: Absolutely.

LEEANN: I'm with you on that.

COACH SHAWN: So, any of the guidelines from your coaches, do you still take advantage of them?

LEEANN: Oh, sure, yeah.

COACH SHAWN: Because you're in...?

LEEANN: I'm on my ninth month right now.

COACH SHAWN: Wow.

LEEANN: Yeah.

COACH SHAWN: You're almost complete.

LEEANN: Yeah, I know. Yeah. So I'm on my ninth month. So I don't really have the one-on-one like you do in the first 120 days. But Karen, my coach, she's like, "Well, we're trying to make it so you're independent and know how to take care of yourself." So she's here for questions, and she is. If I have any questions, I can always contact Dr. Reese too, still, with the ticket system they have.

COACH SHAWN: Do you feel like after those 120 days, you were more self-sufficient?

LEEANN: Yeah, sure, yeah.

COACH SHAWN: That's the value—your life back.

LEEANN: Right. Definitely.

COACH SHAWN: Congratulations on finding peace.

LEEANN: Thank you.

Vertigo Gone, Heart Palpitations Gone, Heart Pain Gone, Digestive Issues Gone

"I finished the 120 program and I'm happy to report that I have healed so many things dramatically. I'm beyond happy. I healed my heart palpitations and heart pain completely. The back pain is mostly gone. PMS is better. My digestion is so much better, I enjoy food for lunch and dinner. I'm just very happy with that. My brain is so much better. I don't have vertigo anymore, no ringing in the ears, I still have some balancing issues but it doesn't bother me much. I can live with it and I enjoy life. Anxiety is better.

A big thank you to Kevin and all the coaches. Thank you doesn't even cover it, what you guys do is life-saving and I'm extremely grateful."

- Lucy

Man Credits Dr. Reese for Life-Changing Recovery from Brain Tumor

"About three years ago, I had a brain tumor the size of a golf ball inside the pituitary region. It was blocking my peripheral vision, and I was losing my sight. If it had continued that way, the tumor would have breached the blood-brain barrier, torn my retina, and left me blind. A host of other complications would have followed. At that time in my life, I was shocked and faced with one of my greatest fears: the prospect of undergoing life-changing brain surgery.

During this challenging period, I began to explore holistic healing approaches, which included a fruit fast. I did a watermelon fast for nearly three months, eating nothing else. While I lost a lot of weight, I also experienced significant healing and prepared my body for the best possible recovery from surgery. The surgeons performed an endoscopic procedure through my nose and into the sphenoid sinus to remove the tumor. Now, three years later, I am completely healed, and it feels as though it never even happened.

I feel incredibly blessed that everything turned out the way it did. This journey changed how I view food and nutrition. Fruit has since become a substantial part of my diet.

After the surgery, I faced a long and challenging recovery. I had lost a significant amount of weight and strength. The drugs, steroids, MRIs, and the surgery itself left me physically depleted. I needed a cane to walk due to poor balance, and I couldn't imagine running or doing any major physical activities. I began physical therapy, stayed committed to a fruit-based diet, and gradually transitioned from eating heavier foods. Through diet, yoga, stretching, and meditation, I began regaining my physical strength and abilities.

For years, I suffered from severe back pain caused by remodeling and flipping homes. I wore a back brace from the moment I woke up until I went to sleep. However, the combination of my surgery, diet, physical therapy, and holistic practices alleviated my back issues. But even with all the progress I made, I eventually reached a plateau. My physical abilities and overall health stagnated, leaving me wondering what I was doing wrong.

Around that time, Dr. Reese introduced his new book, *Peace Over Pain*. Initially, I was unsure whether it would cover new ground or simply revisit concepts I already knew. To my surprise, the book was a revelation. It shed light on the importance of physical balance and the interconnectedness of our muscular and skeletal structures. I realized that limitations in my physical abilities were due to imbalances in my posture and muscular alignment. This insight was transformative.

Locally, I began seeing a physical therapist who specializes in posture therapy, and I now go regularly. Dr. Reese's book made me realize how vital this work is—it's probably more than half the solution for optimal health. Aligning the body not only improves mobility, reduces pain, and builds strength, but it also unlocks energy and vitality. It has given me emotional energy to overcome hurdles I once thought insurmountable.

With better alignment, I've started to stretch more effectively, take yoga more seriously, and meditate without the burden of pain. This, combined with my diet, has allowed me to finally break through those barriers.

I cannot say enough about the holistic approach Dr. Reese has developed. From his guidance on de-stressing to the inner peace fostered through his *Dr. Reese* podcast and the insights in *Peace Over Pain*, he offers a comprehensive formula for healing. His work connects physical, spiritual, and holistic aspects of health in a way that is both practical and deeply personal.

Dr. Reese, thank you for inspiring me to change my life. I admire you and appreciate all the hard work and education you've invested in becoming an example for others. You have truly changed my life. Without your insights, I doubt my brain surgery and recovery would have gone as well as they did. I wish you all the best and hope others discover your meticulous, life-changing work. Much love and peace to you all."

Sciatica Gone in 60 Days, Gums Regenerating, Can Tie Shoes Again

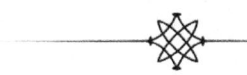

DR. REESE: Angelo, how long did it take for your sciatica and lower back pain to go away?

ANGELO: I would say, okay, since the last time that we had our meeting, maybe two months ago, because that's when I really started getting into my postural therapy. So I would say in two months.

DR. REESE: So two months, and did the sciatica and lower back pain, did it really affect your life?

ANGELO: Well, it did because if it got bad, I couldn't go to work, I couldn't get out of bed, you know, so yeah, it did. For two days, I would have to go to the chiropractor and it would take him about a week to adjust me and, you know, I start to feel better. So yeah, it did affect my life, absolutely. And now it's gone. It's gone, and I've moved my business from one place to another, so I had to do some heavy lifting without a belt, and knock on wood with no pain.

DR. REESE: Wow.

ANGELO: So about a year ago, my bottom gums became loose. It just flapped off, I lost it. Now recently I notice it's starting to grow back.

DR. REESE: Wow.

ANGELO: Yes.

DR. REESE: After 120 days?

ANGELO: After 120 days, yes. I just recently completed my 120th. Yeah. Yeah.

COACH SHAWN: Congratulations.

DR. REESE: What's it like to have discomfort to tie your shoe and then now you don't? It's like something so subtle that nobody thinks about it.

ANGELO: Oh, it's like you don't wanna do it. And it's not only that, if my kids ask me to go play, go run around the backyard with them, I just didn't wanna do it. It's not like I'm tired or anything. I might try to run, I felt like my body wasn't right, you know? It just didn't want to let me do it. I used to want to sit down a lot. If I'm doing nothing, I have to sit down. If I have to tie my kid's shoes, I had to sit down. Now I feel like I notice that I'm standing more up, not sitting down.

DR. REESE: Right on, right. Yes. So subtle.

ANGELO: It's amazing. I'm very happy I joined this program. I'm learning so much.

Low Back Pain Gone

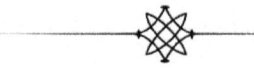

FELICIA: I was in pain this weekend. I went for a 15,000 step walk and I aggravated the hip pain even more. And then on Monday morning I thought, should I do the class, the replay? And so I decided to do it. And then I did Sean's funky move. I don't know what it was. The windmills. It actually helped my pain disappear and I was able to continue to do what I needed to do for the rest of the day. So I really appreciated that. My spine is fused and I have no range of motion. So when I did that particular one, it actually released that pain in my hip.

DR. REESE: Wow. There you go.

FELICIA: So even if you miss a class, the lesson is, do it anyway.

DR. REESE: And this is a great sharing and a great example of healing being a verb. If you go in one direction, it gets better. If you go in the other direction, it gets worse. And so you got to keep going in the right direction. Yeah. That's a great example of that.

COACH SHAWN: Thank you so much for sharing, Felicia. I'm glad it helped with your pain. That's really good to hear.

Debilitating Migraines Gone and Sinus Infections Gone

"I used to get really debilitating migraines, like bad. And now I'm not laid up hiding in hibernation. The sign that everything would be up here because it triggers the sinus infections, everything is all connected. Now I feel like everything is moving. And Coach Connor is awesome.

Like he's got me working. I can see it. And then I lost, I mean, I wasn't trying to lose all this weight, but you know when you eliminate stuff and when your digestive is on point, I lost 10 pounds.

I just feel light as a feather, like I feel so much lighter. It's amazing.

So thank you very much."

Down 30 lbs From Just the Poor 4 Foods!

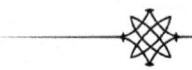

"I got to say, the poor four foods are crazy I'm down like 30 plus now. You know a lot of times it really hurts doing what I do, you know and the joints and everything and Getting off those poor four foods."

Insomnia Gone

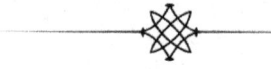

DR. REESE: How has your sleeping changed?

KATIE: Oh, I sleep from 9:30pm to 6am. It's changed drastically. I haven't been able to sleep for the last 10 years, to be honest. And then I got off the medicine and that made it even worse for a while.

KATIE: And I'm six months off the medicine now and I'm just now starting to be able to sleep. And I really credit it to your Insomnia Rescue class. I do the inner child work. I do the postural alignment therapy, and I've been sticking I do the postural alignment therapy. So I really think that's been helpful.

DR. REESE: Very cool.

Hip Pain Gone and Lower Back Pain Gone

DR. REESE: Now, what was it like when you were in the chair and you were in pain, you couldn't get up?

WOMAN: I'd have to kind of wiggle around and get almost some help to get out of the chair. Extreme pain in both hips and lower back. And now I can move!

Neuropathy Gone in 4 Days!?

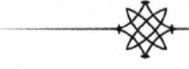

"I just want to give a testimonial to Dr. Kevin Reese. He introduced me to the sugar protocol and once he did that, the feeling in my feet came back within four days and no kidding.

And for those people who are suffering from the onset of neuropathy, you really need to consider talking about this protocol more with Dr. Reese so that you too can feel your feet again."

- Lori T.

Off Thyroid Meds and Lost 30lbs

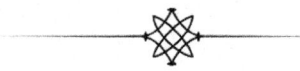

COACH TAMRA: One of our clients, Christine, has graduated, the 120. She's down 30 pounds. She feels good about her relationship with food, so that's good. And her legs have changed a lot. She says they're beautiful now, supposedly, and she can see her knees, so yay!

DR. REESE: Nice, is she here?

CHRISTINE: Hi.

DR. REESE: Hi, Christine. How do you feel about all the changes that you went through?

CHRISTINE: Amazing. I mean, I wish I could tell everybody. I mean, I've told people, but I just don't think they believe. People are not there yet. A lot of people are just not there yet. I think it's amazing.

DR. REESE: Yeah. Your photos. I mean, you're getting cut up.

CHRISTINE: I know. And I'm not even like at the gym. It's in my bedroom on a box.

DR. REESE: You're getting abs.

CHRISTINE: I know.

Interview With Christine

Christine: I had my own blood work done this week, and my thyroid levels were better than ever. That's something I've been battling, and every number came back great.

Dr. Reese: So the program works! Your thyroid is regulating, huh?

Christine: Totally.

Dr. Reese: No meds?

Christine: Nope.

Dr. Reese: Wow. Good for you.

Christine: Thanks.

Dr. Reese: And you were originally on thyroid medication, right?

Christine: Yeah, the synthetic thyroid hormone.

Dr. Reese: How long were you on that before stopping?

Christine: I started taking it in January and stopped around March when I went on the program—whatever year that was. So, not long. But my levels had always been fluctuating. I think the combination of red meat, protein, walking, supplements, and everything else has really made a difference.

Dr. Reese: And postural alignment therapy?

Christine: Yes! Because the thyroid is right here in the neck, right? Our shoulders and neck play a big role in thyroid health.

No Pain Anywhere and Cholesterol Lowered

DR. REESE: How's your progress going?

BLONDIE: Excellent. I couldn't be happier. I have no pain in my body right now. I'm on day 31, I think in the program. The mindfulness training is, I think I'm knocking it out of the park. I think my coach would agree with that. My postural training is awesome. Love it. I'm thrilled. I'm absolutely thrilled. It's really what I was, what I've been looking for for a long long time And I just found it really by luck.

I really did find you by luck on Instagram and it's changed my life, and I'm thrilled. You know, it's not hard. It's not hard. I've done hard things in my life and this is not hard. Yeah. This is just makes sense, you know. Common sense.

DR. REESE: Yeah, it's a great point. It isn't really hard.

BLONDIE: It's not.

DR. REESE: You just follow the road map.

BLONDIE: Yep. I wake up every day in no pain and I love that. It just makes me so happy every day. I get up and I'm like, "I have no pain!".

I know a hundred people who wake up in pain every day, all day long. I do not have pain. And for that, I can't thank you enough. It's wonderful.

"Hi, Dr. Reese. Hi, everyone. My doctor has been dogging me about my cholesterol for a few months now. And, uh, I just ignored the statin that they put in at the pharmacy to, you know, go pick it up. Since I gave up the poor four foods, my cholesterol went down 36 points with no medication. And then my doctor chimed in on my portal and said, um, I still think you need to take the statin."

IBS Gone, Pancreatitis Gone, Ulcers Gone

"So, I was diagnosed with irritable bowel syndrome and stomach ulcers. It made it so I couldn't go about my daily activities. I was always in pain and my stomach was always burning. Every time I ate it was irritating.

They also found that I had a pre-cancerous cyst on my pancreas, so I had to have half my pancreas removed along with my spleen. After surgery every time I ate my pancreas would swell up. I had a lot of pain in that area.

I was always tired all the time, just sluggish, and wasn't myself anymore. I did the Eat the Sunlight program and now I'm full of energy, my pancreas doesn't get swollen anymore. IBS is gone, my ulcer is gone and I feel great."

Fatty Liver Gone, High Blood Pressure Gone, High Cholesterol Gone

"I had high blood pressure, I had high cholesterol and I had fatty liver. The levels were very high and I wasn't feeling good at all. I was fatigued constantly, no matter how much I worked out I was fatigued. I couldn't understand it. The doctor kept telling me that if she doesn't see any changes that she was going to be obligated to give me medication. I kept asking her to give me another chance, give me another chance. After joining Eat the Sunlight, finally after 120 days my liver inflammation went down. The AST level went down sixty points and the ALT levels went down eighty-five points. The blood pressure went down as well, cholesterol went down, I'm energetic, I'm happy and I recommend it." - Maggie

Sciatica Gone

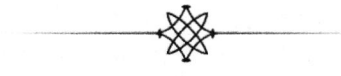

"So for six years, I've been suffering with sciatica pain. Not being able to walk long distances, just out of the blue having pain shoot up my back through my legs. It felt like I couldn't function like I used to. I used to be very active. I used to do kickboxing. I used to jog a lot and I couldn't do a lot of the things that I used to do. So it felt like, you know, a lot of things were changing and I just wasn't myself anymore. It affected being a mom to the point where, you know, when the pain was there, I couldn't really get on the floor and play. I couldn't really take long walks like I used to do with my older son.

I Lost 20 pounds, and most of all, the sciatic pain is gone.

So, even when I think about it these days, like I'm getting ready to go to the park and play with my son, I feel skeptical. I feel like, you know, one day it's gonna just come shooting back, but it's been three months, I haven't had any issues, and it's totally changed my life." - Cateja

Chronic Kidney Dysfunction Gone, Stomach Cramping Gone, High Triglycerides Gone

"For 5 years I suffered from chronic stomach cramping. It felt like someone was twisting my insides and stabbing me constantly.

It changed my life by making me scared to go outside, scared to go to family events, and just constantly scared of eating anything.

I also had chronic kidney dysfunction which affected my life by constantly sending me to the hospital with high fevers and indescribable pain.

Another thing was for over 10 years I had triglycerides and high cholesterol that were out of control. Since doing the program my stomach cramping is completely gone, my kidney dysfunction is gone, my triglycerides dropped over 100 points and my cholesterol is on its way down.

The doctors were completely shocked and I amazed everyone including myself."

- Tara

Running Again...Down 20+ Pounds and Sleeping Great!

"This is my 120-day video. I got the results that I wanted. Those results are less fatigue, less brain fog, I sleep awesome now, I wake up in the morning ready for the day, I love my workouts, I'm running again, And I'm actually enjoying the running. I kept saying to myself that I wasn't going to run again but here I am not only running but setting myself some goals for speed and distance and pushing myself physically again which feels great. Physically I lost a little over 25 pounds."

Sciatica Gone, Acid Reflux Gone, Inflammation Gone, Weight Reduced

COACH SHAWN: Linda's been on the program for a couple of weeks.

LINDA: Sciatica, struggling with that for decades. And that's when I say a huge percentage is gone, I don't wake up with the pain or go to bed with the pain like I used to. It's every once in a while, I'll get a little tinge during the day and I'll go, "what the heck's that?"

It's like now it's a stranger and before it was a constant companion. So that's pretty quick for me because I've tried a lot of other things, but nothing worked. So a lot of inflammation has gone from my body, I can feel it a lot. So I'm super, super happy.

Debilitating Migraines Gone, Off 16 Meds

I used to suffer from migraines. I suffered from that for 14 years. It stopped me from going to work, my daily activity, and that's gone away. There was pressure and a lot of pain in my right side, and I would have to cover my eye and Isolate myself in a dark room, very quiet, and I used to feel the weather coming. Literally, I used to feel the weather coming and tell people there was a storm coming. Everybody hush, hush, be quiet.

Now I don't even get that. Now when the rain comes down, there's thundering, everything, I'm like, "let it rain!"

I'm back to when I was in high school.

Even my neck thinned out, and I lost weight, but that's a bonus. The weight loss is a bonus of healing because I was so swollen from all the prednisone, and a lot of medication.

I can list the names of all my medications because I used to pick them up every month at CVS. Now they're not going to see my face. So they just lost a customer.

Interview With Grissel

Dr. Reese:

This is Dr. Reese, and today it's going to be Griselle vs. Chronic Illness. We're going to talk about her incredible story of 14 years of suffering. I mean, you don't want to miss this. We're talking migraines, we're talking blood pressure, we're talking chronic fatigue, and a whole bunch of other stuff. But now, it's time to talk to Griselle. Hello, Griselle.

Griselle:

Hi, how are you?

Dr. Reese:

Good, great.

Now, all right, you're good now, but my gosh—your story. 14 years of craziness. So let's just start there. What were those 14 years like? Take me back to the pain and the suffering.

Griselle:

Okay, so for 14 years, I was diagnosed... well, prior to the 14 years, I always had headaches—I suffered from headaches. And then 14 years ago, they said, "You know, these are migraines. You're suffering from migraines."

So I would go to one doctor, and that one doctor would send me to another doctor to give me medication. But what would happen is that my body... I couldn't get out of my room. I was very sensitive to lights, to noise. I have children, but back then, I only had three. And it was very difficult for me to actually get up and get out of my house. I isolated myself.

The pain was excruciating. I used to have to hold my right side. I had pressure in my eye. And it was very difficult because I couldn't be part of the social community. I couldn't go out to birthday parties. I constantly had to be locked up, and it actually stopped me from going to work.

I mean, having migraines is very, very hard to handle. It affects your family. It affects you. You get to the point where you're laying in bed for—I mean—four or five hours every afternoon. It makes you very emotional, and then you get other aspects that come into your health, such as depression.

Dr. Reese:

Other kinds of things... So, did the doctors have any clue? Or did they just treat you like a lab rat?

Griselle:

Yes, absolutely. I would go to my primary doctor, and I would get medication for that. Then they sent me to a head specialist, and they gave me more medication. Then they sent me to a sleep doctor, saying it would make things better if I got rest. That didn't make it any better.

Not until I joined *your program*—and I'm going to bring it right there. When I joined *your program* in January of 2017, the first five days, I was waking up, waiting for that pain. I was looking for the pressure in my head, and it wasn't there. But then on the sixth day, seventh day, eighth day, I kept saying, "Oh my God, I don't have any pressure in my head!"

I was so accustomed to waking up with headaches every morning. As it started to get better, I couldn't believe it. I was really functional. I started to be functional—which I hadn't been for so long—and my kids started noticing it.

Dr. Reese:

So, not too long into the program, you started becoming a big-time believer. I remember.

Griselle:

Yeah, yeah, absolutely.

So, having migraines is no joke. It's a very isolating feeling. A lot of people don't understand because they don't suffer from it. But those who do suffer from migraines, they know it's an invisible monster. It just comes in and tackles you. You can't function. You don't want noise, you don't want light, you can't drive. You're sensitive to everything, including a baby crying.

Dr. Reese:

And now your migraines are gone.

Griselle:

Yes, yes, they are. Yes, they are. And I encourage people every time I hear somebody say, "I have a migraine." I tell them, "You guys should join *your program*. You guys don't understand how free you will feel if you just go ahead and join the program."

And sometimes they look at me like I'm a preacher, but no, for real—people need to believe it.

Dr. Reese:

It's hard to make people believe because they were taught something different. It's like telling a five-year-old that Santa Claus isn't real.

Griselle:

You're right. But *your program* is real. I go around telling people all the time.

Every time I hear somebody complain about migraines or fatigue, I tell them, "Oh, you should join *your program*." And they look at me, and I start sharing the beauty of it—the nature of it. Oh my God, I just get emotional. I always get emotional. I feel free. Like, I feel myself again.

It's hard when you feel trapped, and nobody seems to understand your pain. Then they give you one medication for migraines, but that medication gives you constipation. So then they give you another pill for constipation. Now you end up with aches and pains all over your body because you've been trying to push. I'm sorry, but you're in the bathroom trying to handle that.

Now you've got a backache, you sprain your back, you've got to go to the doctor for that. Every time you take medication, it just gives you another complication. And it's awful.

Dr. Reese:

And you were on 16 medications, weren't you? 16?

Griselle:

Yes, yes. I was on 16 different medications.

Because prior to joining *your program*, back in 2011, I was diagnosed with lupus. And with lupus, I also had rheumatoid arthritis and Raynaud's. So there was a lot of medication that came with those symptoms.

But long term, I didn't want to live on medication. And now, I'm not taking any medication. And I feel great. Like, I feel *great*.

I had one doctor say to me, "Oh, keep doing what you're doing." But then I had another doctor—my primary—who said, "We don't see eye to eye."

So it just goes to show you, there are doctors who really care and want you to do better. He commended me because a lot of people get diagnosed, and they just go with the flow. They don't want to do anything about their health. But I decided to make a change.

And my lupus symptoms? They've gotten *so* much better. So much better.

Dr. Reese:

So real quick, let's just confirm this—you're not on any medication right now? Is that what you're saying?

Griselle:

That's correct. That's correct. I was encouraged by one doctor to stay on one medication, which was my methotrexate. He really encouraged me to stay on it, so I tried it for another month. And then I said, "I'm done. I don't need it. I don't feel like I need it. I don't feel sick." So I took myself off medication.

Dr. Reese:

So you went from 16 meds to zero?

Griselle:

Absolutely. And I did it myself, and I let the doctors know. They even put on my report *non-compliant* for my medication intake. So what? I feel better. I eat healthy, I eat clean, I have the stamina that I need, the energy, my kids love me, I'm functional. So I gotta do what I gotta do.

Dr. Reese:

Right.

Now let's go back to a little bit more of the suffering. Your whole body was sore too, right? You had joint pain, nerve pain?

Griselle:

Yes.

Dr. Reese:

And you had high blood pressure?

Griselle:

Yes, I was on medication for that. I was on pain medication for my joints because I used to get inflammation in my knees, ankles, wrists, and shoulders.

At one point, I was getting therapy for my shoulder. The doctors suggested I should get rotator cuff therapy because otherwise, I would need surgery. I don't even have that issue anymore.

Look, I mean, I exercise, I eat well... but being sick is hard. People don't understand. You can't go out and shop for yourself. You can't even push a shopping cart at the grocery store. You have to run out because your body is achy. You don't even have the drive to leave your house. You don't want to get out of your pajamas when you're sick.

Now, I'm up at 4:30–5:00 in the morning like a little rabbit.

Dr. Reese:

Right, right.

Griselle:

I mean, it's tough being sick. People don't understand. Medication doesn't really help. It just helps at the moment with the actual symptom, but then you get it again. And then you get it again. And then again.

People don't understand that medication is *not* a solution. That's not getting to the root cause of the problem. And that's what I said when I first joined *your program*. I didn't want to keep covering up my symptoms. I didn't want to cover up my pain. I wanted it to go away. And it did. And it did. I want everybody to know—it did.

Dr. Reese:

Yeah, your migraines went away fast. Migraines always go away fast in this program—usually within six weeks.

Griselle:

Yeah. I started feeling different because I had an aneurysm, and it got clipped.

We followed it, and it was pretty big. They told me, "On June 6th, 2014, you're going to have to get a clip." And at first, I was very nervous because the neurosurgeons told me, "50% of your body may not function after surgery."

So I put it in God's hands. I said, "You know what? God is almighty. I have children. I need to go through this."

Sure enough, I went through it. And after surgery, my migraines became so bad that when I had a heavy migraine, my right eye would go blurry.

So I went to an ophthalmologist. The ophthalmologist said, "You're fine, you can see."

I said, "No, I can't." Because when I covered my good eye, I saw like I had a… like a booger. I'm sorry, but I really felt like I had mucus covering my eye.

But now, I can see clearly. I can look left, I can look right. Dr. Reese, I can see! I feel great. It's *different*.

Dr. Reese:

Do you think the brain surgery had a lot to do with them testing different medications on you—kind of that whole lab rat type of thing?

Griselle:

You know, I don't know. Because they kept giving me different medications for the migraines.

I mean, one doctor said to me, "You shouldn't really be on that Brutal medication because it's not going to let you sleep."

But then they gave me medication for sleeping, which was Ambien. They said, "Here you go."

And then the sleep doctor said, "Because you have anxiety, you can't sleep. Here's Clonazepam."

So, I mean, I can say all their names because they kept trying different medications on me. And I just felt like they just wanted to see me every six weeks.

Different specialty teams wanted to see me—like a membership program.

Dr. Reese:

Right.

Griselle:

They just wanted to keep seeing me. And it was hard.

Now it's like, "Oh, we'll see you in a year."

Dr. Reese:

Right.

Now let's talk about the lupus. Typically, when you get lupus, it always stays on your record, even if the symptoms go away. They call it remission, right? Kind of like cancer—"My cancer is in remission, my lupus is in remission."

Where are you now with your lupus? What are your symptoms now?

Griselle:

Well, right now, from all the symptoms that I had…

Mind you, when I was first diagnosed with lupus, I had a big bald spot on my head because I was losing my hair. That was one of the first symptoms.

My second symptom was cold extremities—real frozen extremities. That symptom I still have. My fingertips and toes still get cold. Even when I exercise, even if I'm in the sauna.

But other than that, my fatigue is gone. My blood pressure is gone. My energy is up. So a lot of my symptoms have diminished.

Like the whole list of criteria they say you have to meet for lupus—I don't meet those anymore.

But like I said, it was one of those invisible monsters. You don't know when you're going to get a symptom.

But I haven't had one, except for the Raynaud's.

From all the other symptoms I used to have—joint pain, ankle swelling—I mean, I'm telling you, it's awesome. It's awesome to feel this way.

So I'm still working on it, but it's cold now, so I know that takes time.

Dr. Reese:

It's going to take time.

Griselle:

It's going to take time because it took time for me to get sick. All those years of eating foods that I didn't know were harming me. It took time for my body to break down, so it's going to take some time to heal.

But I feel like I'm at 98%.

Dr. Reese:

Right.

You're coming up on a year.

Griselle:

Yes, I am.

Dr. Reese:

You know, this is just a prediction from me, but I'd say once you hit two full years, you're going to be *completely* fine. That's my prediction. If you continue, which I believe you will.

Griselle:

Yes. Yes, I will.

This is a *lifestyle*. If people think this is a diet program, it's not a diet program. It's not a weight-loss program. This is a *lifestyle change*.

And it's for those who want to be healthy, strong, and live a *quality* life.

Dr. Reese:

You love those medicinal teas. You're always ordering tea.

Griselle:

I love them! Because if I have a hard time sleeping, I take the tea.

I actually posted the other day—it was like one something in the morning—I took some, and I went to bed. It took me maybe about an hour, but at least I wasn't just sitting there.

Dr. Reese:

Did you take the Anxiety Tea or the Sleep Helper?

Griselle:

No, I took the Sleep Helper. And it worked! I like the taste of it, too.

I also do the Anxiety Tea. I don't have to take medication for that anymore—I feel better.

Even one of my biggest concerns was when I had to take my twins to the doctor and advocate for their needs. I used to get really flustered. My thought process would get thrown off because I had to keep explaining to adults what was wrong with my children or what their needs were, and they just didn't seem to understand.

That's when my anxiety would kick in.

But since I've been on the tea, I actually feel *a lot* calmer. I just keep smiling at people—like, *if only they knew*.

Dr. Reese:

It's like magic.

Griselle:

They don't know who they're dealing with now! If someone had spoken to me a certain way a year and a half ago, I would have responded *completely* differently.

With all those medications, you get mood swings. Your attitude changes so bad.

Dr. Reese:

Now, Griselle, I remember you came to a small little seminar I did with Tina. I believe it was in Glastonbury, back in 2014, when I released my book.

I remember you from that day—you were sick. Did you leave that room different, or did you think, "Oh, this guy's just a quack job. He's crazy"?

Griselle:

No, I left *different*. I really left different.

I was telling Tina, "I love this. I love this!" We got the book. I was reading it. I got *excited*.

I just didn't know how to jump into the program at the time. I didn't know how to start leaving my meat behind.

But it *felt* good. I said, *This is going to be me. This is going to be me.*

You have to *want* it.

Then when Tina told me, "Kevin has these medicinal teas," I said, "Well, let's do it."

Because if I had been trusting doctors all this time—taking medication, going through the same cycle with no healing, just covering things up, a temporary fix—why not try this?

And look, I'm so *glad* I did.

I encourage *everybody* to do it.

I go around constantly telling people.

When I hear people whining—because you know what? I call it whining, because I *was* a whiner too.

I used to whine, "It hurts, it hurts, it hurts! Don't bother me, don't talk to me."

Now I'm like, "You *can* be happier. You *really* can, if you just try this."

Dr. Reese:

Yeah, you do go about it differently. You have to *change* your lifestyle.

Griselle:

Yes.

Dr. Reese:

Now, let's go back again.

You said you weren't able to go to your family get-togethers. And you have *seven* children, right?

Griselle:

Yes.

Dr. Reese:

And grandkids?

Griselle:

I have seven grandbabies—two biological, and three step-grandkids that my daughter is raising.

And they *always* have functions.

Dr. Reese:

And you're Puerto Rican, too.

Griselle:

Yes, I am! And I don't need no pork.

I don't need no pork, I don't need no rice, I don't need *none* of that nonsense.

Dr. Reese:

Boricuas love to party—family parties.

Griselle:

Yes!

Dr. Reese:

So I *know* there were tons of events you missed over those years.

Griselle:

Yeah. Absolutely.

Dr. Reese:

Did your family get on you about it?

Griselle:

Yes. It was very hard.

I was called a party pooper. "You're always ruining things. Come on, you can do it."

They couldn't *understand* what was happening in my body.

They were so *mean*.

And that's when depression kicks in—because you feel like you're letting them down.

You've got the *guilt* of being sick. You start asking, "Why me? Why did this happen to *me*?"

And then you see family pictures... pictures you *should* have been in... and I get emotional.

Because I should have been there. But my *body* wouldn't let me be out there.

Dr. Reese:

Right.

Griselle:

My body was *controlling* me.

And a lot of people don't understand.

I had to leave my job—one of the best jobs, too, that I *loved*—working with kids in the school system.

Because I couldn't get up in the morning.

I would wake up stiff, in pain.

Sometimes, I would call the secretary and say, "Oh, Miss So-and-So, I'm not able to come to work."

And she'd go, "What is it *now*? Your *ear*?"

Like, so cruel.

People don't *understand*—when you have lupus or when you have a migraine attack, my migraines would last *seven, eight, nine* straight days.

It wasn't like, "Oh, I'll take a pill and it'll go away."

No.

They would *drug* me up to put me to sleep. I'd sleep for five, six hours, wake up... and it was *still* there.

The next day? Same cycle.

So, I missed a *lot* of family events. A *lot* of community events that I loved participating in.

And now, when I look at pictures from those times, I think, *Wow... I missed so much when I was sick.*

Dr. Reese:

And now? Now you're able to go out there.

Now you're able to go to those functions, you're bouncing around Hartford, telling *everyone* about *your program*, you can go to your family events...

How does your family treat you *now*?

Because now you're able to *come*—but you're *not* eating exactly how they're eating. So now, it's like another layer.

Griselle:

Yeah, they tell me, "Oh, that's *cute*."

Now, when I go, the first thing they say is, "Oh, you're on a diet! That's right, you don't eat."

I say, "No. I am *not* on a diet. I'm on a *new lifestyle*. I want to *stay* healthy. This is what I'm doing."

But I *still* contribute.

I walk in with a beautiful salad. I decorate it really nice. Or I bring a fruit salad when I go to functions.

I'm still as silly as ever.

But when I was sick? I *wasn't* silly. I was like a bitter woman because I didn't have the drive. I didn't *want* to go anywhere.

Now that I go places, they *really* enjoy me being there.

But they'll still say, "Oh, come on, you can have *some* pork. You can have a little *pernil*."

And I tell them, "I'm not going to get sick again."

Dr. Reese:

And I tell them, "I'm not going to get sick again."

Griselle:

And I tell them, "Here, take a look at this." I hand them a brochure. I tell them about *your program*, about the tea, about everything.

I show them my display.

And a couple of them say, "Tell me more."

You know what *really* frustrates me, though?

When I tell them about it, and they say, "I'll get to it."

I say, "*Let's do it now!* If you're really serious, do it *now*! The change is *today*! It's not tomorrow. It's *right now*."

And that's how I got a few people to join. You know a lot of my girlfriends joined.

I tell them, "*Right now* is the moment. If you're really serious about your health and you want to live a *quality* life, do it *now*."

Dr. Reese:

Yeah, you did get a few people in.

Griselle:

Eileen.

Dr. Reese:

Your childhood friend.

Griselle:

Eileen, yes.

And Madeline.

Dr. Reese:

Madeline, that's right.

Griselle:

Benita did, too.

Dr. Reese:

You know, I was just telling someone the other day that it's *harder* to convince people of the *idea* than it is to convince them to spend the money.

Because people just *can't* believe it.

Like I said, they weren't *brought up* with this knowledge.

This is real *science*, but it's been suppressed.

And it's going to take *time* for people to start waking up.

For example, two years ago, the *World Health Organization*—not America, *World* Health Organization—came out and said that *processed meats contribute to cancer.*

That's a *bold* statement. It had never been said before.

But it only made the news *for one day*.

You know what I mean? It was only on the news *that day*.

Nobody's talking about it *now*.

It wasn't reinforced in the human mind. So, what happens? People keep eating their hot dogs, their salami, their sausage, their bacon—because they *don't know any better*.

Nobody's telling them *not to*.

Sure, here and there, a Netflix documentary will come out. Maybe they'll run into someone like me on Instagram or Facebook.

But they have *no clue*.

So when they see *you*—so excited, so passionate—they just look at you like, *Okay... what's this new club she's in? Is this a cult? What new religion is she into?*

People are just *scared* of newness.

And it's going to take *time*, Griselle. Wouldn't you say?

Griselle:

It's going to take *time*.

But as we keep seeing results, and as more people start joining, and as we stay *true* to the program and this *lifestyle*, people are going to realize—

"Wait a minute... I know her. She used to be sick. Now look at her."

Because my friends and family *know* me.

And when *they* start getting sick—when *they* end up on all these medications—when *they* have all these symptoms that won't go away—

That's when they're going to say, "*I don't want to be sick anymore.*"

And my *hope* is that they don't have to hit rock bottom first.

I *hope* they don't have to go through all the suffering I went through.

But *some* people *need* to hit rock bottom before they wake up.

And that's why it's important that you keep doing what you do.

So you can keep educating people.

And you have people like *me* spreading the message.

Dr. Reese:

Right.

Griselle:
I'm *so* excited about the program.

Dr. Reese:

I *know* you are. I *know* you are.

And I *really* appreciate that passion.

How do you feel when you see someone else come out of the program with results?

Griselle:

I feel *great*!

I feel *so* happy!

Because everyone has *different* results, right? Everyone's healing journey is different.

But I've noticed something—

A *common* thing that *everybody* seems to have before joining... is *migraines*.

I was thinking the other day...

Could migraines also be triggered by all these different medications?

Because *so many* people have migraines. Like, *severe* migraines.

And I bet you—it's probably the *side effects* of all these medications mixing together in people's systems.

Dr. Reese:

That's a *good* observation, Griselle.

Because if you look at the data from *your program*, migraines *always* go away.

Everyone who comes in with migraines or headaches—*they don't have them anymore after six weeks*.

Griselle:

That's right.

Dr. Reese:

And blood pressure is the other big one.

Blood pressure and migraines—those two things? They go away *fast*.

Griselle:

Yes!

So for people out there who *just* have migraines...

If they can't function—if they have to call out of work all the time—if migraines are affecting their *income*—

This should be the number one program they join.

Because once they get rid of their migraines, they'll be *functional*.

They won't have to call out sick. They won't have to lay in bed all day.

And *this* is the way to do it.

And I *learned* that.

And now—I'm *free*.

I'm *free* from migraines.

I'm *free* from fatigue.

Dr. Reese:

You *are* the walking billboard.

Griselle:

I'm *free*!

Dr. Reese:

You *are* the walking billboard.

Griselle:

And I'm Puerto Rican!

We're *supposed* to be eating all the pork and the rice and the pasteles.

But guess what?

We *don't need it*.

We can *survive* without it.

Dr. Reese:

And you lost weight, too.

Griselle:

Yes!

I lost *63 pounds* already!

So it's *good*. It's *awesome*.

I grew my hair back.

There are *so many* positive things.

Dr. Reese:

Yeah.

Awesome.

Well, keep up the great work, and keep spreading the word.

It's a *mission*. It's *missionary work*.

People *need* to know about this.

So you're a *great* mouthpiece for that.

You're an *inspiration* to a lot of people.

And let me ask you—does it make you feel good when someone says, *"You inspire me"*?

Griselle:

Yes! Yes, it does.

It makes me feel *great*.

And I love the *other* program you have—the Anxiety program.

I love the tips you share.

Like learning how to *breathe*—that has *helped* me so much.

I think I used to *hyperventilate* every time I got worked up.

Now, I know how to *breathe*—four in, hold for four, four out.

I do that multiple times a day, and I feel *so* good.

Dr. Reese:

Right.

Griselle:

Yeah, different avenues.

Dr. Reese:

Absolutely.

Well, *thank you* for taking the time to share your incredible story.

14 years of suffering—that's a *long* time.

Griselle:

Yes.

Head To Toe Healing

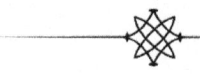

As you have read from these amazing testimonials, HEAD TO TOE HEALING is your answer. If you don't get going on your healing journey, you could and will end up in a dark place.

The harsh reality is that the medical monopoly is not trained to heal you, they are trained to treat your symptoms, stabilize you and manage your pain with drugs, injections and surgeries.

In order to prove my new practice of HEAD TO TOE HEALING, I have captured the results on camera. People from all over the world on camera testifying to multiple symptoms disappearing.

This is confusing to many people because they have been brainwashed by the medical monopoly to need the help of specialists. You know, the spine specialist, the brain specialist, the GI specialist, the mental health specialist, the foot specialist and so on.

Well, my speciality is the whole body!

It's probably going to take another 100 years for people to truly understand HEAD TO TOE HEALING because people are so programmed to ask about their diabetes, or tinnitus, or bunions, or fibromyalgia, or migraines, or herniated disks etc that they lose sight of the truth.

The truth is...your body is a whole unit.

If there's something wrong with your feet, I want to see your ears. If there's something wrong with your ears, I want to see your feet. It's all connected.

HEAD TO TOE HEALING is the opposite of the medical monopoly specialist, it's about zooming out and viewing the body as a whole unit. Then we want to put it back into its natural alignment so that it heals. You see, the body is divinely designed to heal itself. God set it up this way!

To further understand how to perform HEAD TO TOE HEALING, I've broken the body down into 3 categories.

1. You have a vehicle (musculoskeletal system)
2. You need proper fuel for the vehicle (nutrition)
3. There's an onboard computer that runs the vehicle (the mind)

So if you have a pain in your left knee...

It could be coming from misalignments of your musculoskeletal system...

Or it could be coming from improper nutrition...

Or it could be coming from a lack of mindfulness...

It also could be coming from all three!

It doesn't matter because with the method of HEAD TO TOE HEALING, it's about getting after all three sections of the body, no matter what!

We approach type 2 diabetes the same way we approach a herniated disk, it's the same practice.

There's no over-diagnosis and there's no over-treatment with drugs, injections or surgeries.

You begin by ordering your HEAD TO TOE Analysis so that I can see the alignment of feet, knees, hips, shoulders, spine, neck and skull. Along with your nutritional profile and mental health status, you walk away with the root causes of your symptoms that a medical professional couldn't give you. This will give you the "ah-ha" moment that you needed to truly understand HEAD TO TOE HEALING. You also receive your "symptom score" which acts as a gauge to your health status.

Once you're evaluated and have a symptom score, you can enter my HEAD TO TOE HEALING Membership where you can come to our daily livestreams and start your 120 day program. This infamous program jumpstarts your HEAD TO TOE HEALING journey by getting after the whole body strategically.

So for example, if you scored a 30 on your analysis and your score at the end of 120 days is a 15, you're moving in the right direction. You're HEAD TO TOE HEALING.

Keep in mind, healing is a verb, it's a process, it's a moving thing which is why there can be no absolute "cure." Let the medical monopoly have the word "cure" we are HEAD TO TOE HEALING.

If you wish to learn more about my new method, it's important that you read or listen to my entire book collection.

You can purchase these books here:

https://www.drkevinreese.com/books

Q & A
WITH DR. REESE

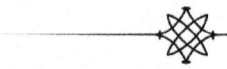

I'M ON STATIN DRUGS AND MY MUSCLES HURT. HOW DO I GET OFF THESE STUPID DRUGS!?

If I were you, I would simply just stop. Statins have no addictive quality to them and don't not need a weaning process. If you'd like to play it safe, you can cut your dose in half for a few weeks and then stop. The reason you're having cramps is because the drugs have created a cholesterol deficiency in your body. Cholesterol is a very important nutrient that nourishes soft tissue. Muscle is soft tissue, organs are soft tissue, glands are soft tissue, eyes are soft tissue and most certainly, your brain is soft tissue. That's why most people that have been on statins for decades end up with dementia.

I HAVE TINNITUS? WHAT DO I DO? I'M GOING INSANE.

You do HEAD TO TOE HEALING. There's so many reasons why you could have this ringing in your ear that they call tinnitus. Is it the position of your neck? Is it a nutritional deficiency? Is it osteoporosis of the skull? Is it a blood sugar issue? The beautiful thing about HEAD TO TOE HEALING is it doesn't matter that much. You get after your whole body and let it do its work. Don't focus on the symptom, instead focus on your entire body. I suggest you order a HEAD TO TOE ANALYSIS and then get into the membership and you'll be on your way. If you view our testimonies, you'll see tinnitus disappear quite a few times.

IS THERE A CERTAIN WAY I SHOULD SLEEP SO I DON'T MESS UP MY POSTURE?

The answer is yes and no. Laying flat on your back is always the best way to rest. However, sleep is so important that you should sleep however you can. I would rather you get 8 hours in the fetal position than 3 hours on your back. So sleep however you can. This is why we do PAT (postural alignment therapy) in my membership. PAT is to your muscles what brushing and flossing is to your teeth. Your muscles need to be maintained daily. Also, as soon as you wake up, banging out some cats & dogs is ideal.

THEY TOOK MY GALLBLADDER! NOW WHAT?

Well, unfortunately, the medical monopoly doesn't tell you what to do. They just cut you and then sent you on your way right? So I'll tell you right now that you need to be on enzymes with ox bile for the rest of your life. You're now handicapped and need a crutch. I'll also tell you a harsh reality, you probably didn't need your gallbladder taken out. They are notorious for overdiagnosing. I have a course in my membership called Gallbladder Rescue that has helped many reverse their situation. Just know that the root causes that triggered your gallbladder are still there. It's like a shark circling the boat but you can't see the fin. You need HEAD TO TOE HEALING before more symptoms hit you.

I HEAR THAT ALL DISEASE COMES FROM THE GUT? IS IT TRUE?

No. This is a fun statement that health practitioners make because they are not HEAD TO TOE HEALERS yet. Certainly, the gut didn't cause your bunion or your herniated disk right? What they mean to say is that the gut is a root cause of most biochemical diseases. You see, muscle dysfunction is the root cause of most musculoskeletal misalignments (posture) which can also mess up the gut. Right in back of the gut is a spine and the position of that spine matters for gut health. Furthermore, the mind can give you gut symptoms. Understanding the body from HEAD TO TOE is a rare thing. Everything is connected.

HOW CAN I ORDER THE PROPER BLOOD LABS MYSELF WITHOUT MY PHYSICIAN? AND DOES INSURANCE COVER IT?

Inside my membership, we show you where to go, how to order and how to read the labs yourself. You can even order my recommended labs which cover most of your nutritional profile. Once you order, you can go to your local Quest or Labcorp to have the blood drawn and your results will be sent to your Quest or Labcorp phone app. It's not covered by insurance and that's a good thing. By paying out of pocket you are taking your control back and becoming independent. I'm teaching you how to save yourself and not be reliant on a corrupt system.

DR REESE, I'M SO DEPRESSED, I DON'T EVEN WANT TO GET UP IN THE MORNING. WHAT CAN I DO?

Make high pitched noises. Start there. This will elevate your frequency. Look at the word itself. It says that you're being pressed downward. So let's go upward! Furthermore, you need to make sure you don't have a nutritional deficiency. Missing one nutrient can cause up to 10 symptoms, so that's 900 total. Certainly, one of those symptoms could be depression. So getting on the right supplements is key. Of course, you have to get off the poor four foods (gluten, oils, friend and fake). You also could have a compressed nerve that alters your moods. However, the usual cause of depression is a lack of mindfulness. Many people get stuck in their heads and have a very negative voice talking in there. This creates disappointment and hopelessness. This is your inner child talking. In my membership, I teach my people how to work with the inner child to deprogram, reprogram and heal. The result will make you happy and appreciative.

WHAT TYPE OF WATER SHOULD I DRINK?

Well, not tap water. A RO (reverse osmosis) system is probably the most convenient way to filter water because once you install it you can drink it, cook with it, wash dishes with it and wash off food with it. Just make sure when you drink it, you re-mineralize. I also like the Berkey filtering system because it doubles as a mobile emergency unit. In other words, if your city's water becomes contaminated, you can find a local stream or pond and filter it through your Berkey unit. Hydrogen water is the new craze and it can help hydrate you perhaps better than any other water. As far as bottled water, it's best if you stay away from flimsy plastic because chemicals can leach into the water. Hard plastic is a better option and glass is the best option. Lastly, always stay away from carbonated and alkaline water, it decreases your stomach acid levels and will eventually cause acid reflux.

MY DENTIST SAYS I NEED A ROOT CANAL. SHOULD I GET IT DR. REESE?

If I were you, I wouldn't do it. There have been so many people who end up with health issues after this procedure. I have a course in my membership called Mouth Rescue. In there I will educate you on how to fix your mouth.

WHAT DO I DO ABOUT PARASITES?

Top off on stomach acid! Parasites only exist inside you if you don't have proper stomach acid (unless you're in a jungle). This is why so many vegans and plant based people have parasites. They detox out their worms and then show it off on social media which makes everyone paranoid that they have an infestation inside of them. The whole reason they had the worms in the first place is because they have low stomach acid and that acid is low because they've been obsessed with alkalizing. They're not HEAD TO TOE HEALERS and don't understand the full scope of the body. You need a stomach acid level that is comparable to battery acid. Stomach acid deficiency is a root cause of a lot of symptoms, that's why we test it in our HEAD TO TOE Analysis.

WHERE ARE YOU LOCATED?

It doesn't matter. We are 100% virtual and help people from all over the world. We have people in my membership from the USA, UK, Australia, New Zealand, Portugal, South Africa and more. The only time to actually see me in person is at my annual seminar every spring. It's always held in my home state of Connecticut, USA. It's a great opportunity to not only meet me, but the rest of the membership. It's like a family reunion.

MY SISTER HAS AFIB AND IT'S DRIVING HER NUTS! WHAT CAN I DO TO HELP?

First off, you can't do anything except pass on information. She has to save herself. I would suggest the MEDICAL MONOPOLY and or PEACE OVER PAIN books. Give it to her and see if she wakes up. Please understand, AFib is typically a compressed nerve in the spine due to a musculoskeletal misalignment (posture). Then again, it could also be a nutritional deficiency. Does it matter? If your sister wakes up and does HEAD TO TO HEALING the chances of her AFib going away is very high.

SO YOU DON'T GO TO A DOCTOR?

I don't. I take care of myself through the practice of HEAD TO TOE HEALING. I pay out of pocket to run blood work once or twice per year just like I teach you in my membership. I do my PAT (postural alignment therapy), I take my supplements, I stay away from the poor four foods, I get 10,000 steps per day and I practice my mindfulness training. If something happens that requires medical attention, then I go to the nearest Urgent Care Center and pay a few hundred bucks. If something really serious happens, then I would use my health sharing program to pick up the tab for the ER. By not having a doctor I am claiming my freedom and adopting a HEAD TO TOE HEALING mindset. This is what I'm teaching you.

I HAVE FEET PAIN. WHAT SHOULD I DO?

Feet are at the mercy of your pelvis. When your pelvis is tilted, rotated or elevated it will affect the way you walk around earth (gait pattern). The more you walk a certain way the more your feet take a beating. Before you know it you may develop hammertoes, calluses or a bunion forming. We have a course in my membership called Foot Rescue that will move you in the right direction.

WHY DO YOU TALK SO SLOW AND WEIRD? IT'S CREEPY!

I'm working on different levels. One level I'm giving you health information so that you may heal yourself. On another level, I'm talking in a soft and calm way so that it may relax you from your busy life. On another level, I'm leaving space in between my words so that you can get to the spaciousness that's available to you. On another level, I'm putting out an energy that only those that are open can tap into. My style of communicating is not for everyone and that's good. If someone finds it creepy or weird, then I am not for them. They're not ready to be with me. Not everyone will understand what I have just said to you.

I AM ON 23 MEDICATIONS AND I FEEL TRAPPED!

You're in medical prison! This is the result of trusting in people that aren't trained to heal you. If you want to escape the prison, you have a long road ahead of you. If I were you, I would get off of any statin drugs or PPIs (proton pump inhibitors) because these are the two medications that are counteractive. In other words, you can't really perform HEAD TO TOE HEALING with them in your system. Next, get off the poor four foods (gluten, oils, fried and fake). Use my cookbook for recipes if you need to. Lastly, keep watching my videos. That's it. Start there because you're so programmed and traumatized right now that your inner child doesn't know who to trust! These three changes I just gave you will serve you well. Give it 60 days and I believe that you're going to feel major improvements. After you feel the changes and the faith has been established, come back and order an analysis. Then the next step is getting you into my membership and the journey of HEAD TO TOE HEALING will truly begin.

ARE YOU A KIND OF LIKE A CHIROPRACTOR?

No. Chiropractors are specialists in the alignment of the skeletal system. They snap, crackle and pop you with physical manipulation. In HEAD TO TOE HEALING we focus on the whole body (all 11 systems) and we don't have to lay a hand on you. That's how we have a virtual membership with people HEAD TO TOE HEALING from all over the world. People confuse me with a chiropractor because I'm talking about "alignment" all the time. The chiropractors kind of own that word just like the medical monopoly owns "diagnose," "treat" and "cure."

HOW DO I GET MY CHILDREN AWAY FROM THE HARMFUL JUNK FOODS?

Well, if they're under the age of 5 then I have a solution. I created a children's project based around a superhero named, SUNLIGHT SONNY. He flies all around the world helping kids stay away from the evil, Mr. Junkerson and his junk food. There's books, music and an animated TV show. However, if the kids are over 5, you have to just be repetitive and keep making them understand. A little trick you can pull if you're ok with a white lie, is telling your child that they're allergic to the poor 4 foods (gluten, oils, fried and fake). It works! I mean, most parents are already lying about Santa Clause anyway. You may be saving their future.

WHAT DO YOU THINK IS THE DISEASE THAT MOST AFFECTING SOCIETY?

Brain conditions, hands down. Everyone is scared of the C-Monster but it's dementia (Alzheimer's, FTD and Lewy body), parkinsons, ALS and MS that are making the biggest impact. How can we have a society when people's brains are compromised? A brain condition essentially takes you right out of the work force and puts you on the disability list. It's so preventable. It's a sad story.

WHAT DO YOU THINK OF THE CARNIVORE DIET?

I like the carnivore diet as a protocol. It's a great way to counteract conditions such as SIBO or Diabetes. However, I don't like the idea of being on this diet for longer than 90 days. Nutrition is based on ratios and all muscle meat is low in calcium and high in phosphorus which can trigger the body to steal calcium from the bones, teeth and nails. Therefore, someone that wanted to stay on Carnivore should be supplementing, as should everyone in the modern world. It's important to note that humans are meant to eat the whole animal, nose to tail, which would contain every nutrient needed. However, humans don't eat the whole animal anymore, they just like muscle meat.

I'VE SEEN YOUR ANALYSIS ON BRUCE LEE AND NOW I'M WORRIED THAT I ALSO MAY HAVE FORWARD HEAD. HOW CAN I FIND OUT?

First, thank you for paying attention to my videos. Second, in order to discover the position of your neck and head you would order a HEAD TO TOE Analysis. That way, I can evaluate your entire body, not just your head. Forward head, as you know now, is a problem in society. Once that neck starts falling out onto the chest, it's going to create "above the shoulder" symptoms. This could be ringing in the ears, dizziness, chronic headaches, eye issues, mouth issues and more. It could even contribute to dementia or parkinsons in the future. The reason why is because the lymphatic fluid in the head can't drain properly. Also, the blood and oxygen can't flow up to the brain, eyes, ears, nose and mouth as well.

SO YOU'RE SAYING I SHOULDN'T GET MY MAMMOGRAM?

If I were you, I would never have anything scanned unless I actually had symptoms (in this case a lump). Secondly, I would have it checked through Thermography. It's a very simple gray scan that can show lumps forming. It's important to note that if you do have a lump, you're still going to be faced with the medical monopolies only three solutions; drugs, injections or surgery. Perhaps I'm biased, but I feel that HEAD TO TOE HEALING is a better option due to the fact that the cause of the symptom(s) has to do with the whole body. The medical monopoly is just going to "zoom in" on the issue and throw the baby out with the bathwater.

HOW DO I BECOME AS CALM AS YOU DR. REESE?

It took me a very long time to evolve into the calm and peaceful man you see. Mindfulness training over and over and over again. It took a lot of failing. Luckily, I feel I have condensed the teachings and made it easier for you. You shouldn't have to go through as tough a time as I went through. In my membership, I'll teach you how to work with your inner child to move toward peace and healing. However, I do have a cheat code. It's the formula of acceptance + appreciation =

inner peace. You see, most people have emotional imbalance because they don't accept life, therefore, they resist it in their head. They like the good of life but reject the bad and the ugly of life. Secondly, most people don't appreciate what they already have, including the hard times which are essentially lessons. For example, let's say you come out of the grocery store and your car window is smashed! What an inconvenience right? Well, accept it. Why wouldn't your window get smashed? It's a window! Also, appreciate that you even have a car to begin with. You know, some people take the bus. Also, appreciate the lesson that is being taught to you. Wait, what's the lesson? Find it, learn from it, smile, laugh and move on.

WAIT, YOU'RE NOT A MEDICAL DOCTOR?

That's correct. I'm a fake doctor. Dr. Reese is my stage name...kinda like Dr. Dre.

I HAVE HIGH CHOLESTEROL, WHAT SHOULD I DO TO CONTROL IT?

Nothing. In HEAD TO TOE HEALING, cholesterol is your friend and you don't want to try to control it. You need cholesterol to nourish your soft tissue. I would be more concerned with your Triglycerides and CRP levels as it pertains to cardiovascular health. You have been programmed to be scared of cholesterol, but it's not your enemy. You can read more about it in my book, REVERSE THE CAUSE and or there's a webinar I made for you on it on my website.

I HEAR ALOT ABOUT MOVING THE LYMPHATIC SYSTEM THESE DAYS. WHAT SAY YOU?

It's important. The lymphatic system is the sewage system of the body and it eliminates cellular waste from the body. Sometimes it can become clogged up from tight clothes, lack of exercise or from musculoskeletal misalignment. You want your lymph to be like a river and not like a pond. In my membership, we have three PAT (postural alignment therapy) classes per week. Not only will this get your musculoskeletal system back in alignment, but it will move your lymph. You see, the lymphatic system doesn't have a pump so it relies on your joints to act as a pumping system. You also need the "highways" to be open, so that's where something like tight clothes or muscle dysfunction slows things down. If the lymph slows down, many symptoms can occur, including tumors, nodules, cysts and polyps. In my membership, we also have a course called Lymph Rescue.

HOW CAN I MAKE AN APPOINTMENT WITH YOU DR. REESE?

I don't do personal appointments. Meeting with the "doctor" is an outdated strategy based on you feeling comfortable that an expert is there for you. I would rather you be uncomfortable and go on a journey to learn how to save yourself. If you're interested then go to www.DREKEVINREESE.com and poke around. When you're ready, make an appointment with my coaching team to see if HEAD TO TOE HEALING is the right fit for you. Remember, only you can save you.

WHY ARE OILS IN YOUR POOR FOUR FOODS? DO YOU JUST MEAN SEED OILS? THERE SEEMS TO BE SO MANY BENEFITS OF OLIVE OIL!

I teach my people to stop eating all oil, including olive oil. This is due to the fact that the oil has been pressed from the whole food. Now, this fat juice is vulnerable to oxidation from the air. Once that happens, the oil becomes rancid and free radicals are formed. Of course this creates free radical damage (oxidative stress) in the body which is a root cause for cardiovascular dis-ease and the C-Monster. If you go find a bottle of oil right now, you will notice space at the top of the bottle. In other words, the bottle isn't filled all the way up. What's in that space at the top? Right, it's oxygen. How long was the oil bathing in the oxygen? Hours? Days? Months? Now your salad is a weapon of mass destruction. Even worse, if you cook the oil, you've just made it even more destructive and you have set yourself up for a really ugly health event in the future. If you don't want to cook with water (that's how I cook) then use butter, ghee, lard or tallow like your ancestors did.

HAVING NO HEALTH INSURANCE SOUNDS SCARY, WHY ARE YOU RECOMMENDING THIS?

So that you can unplug from the medical monopoly and be independent. Of course it's a case by case thing. If you're stuck in MEDICAL PRISON then you have to have insurance. However, if you're a healthy person, why would you? Especially if you're practicing HEAD TO TOE HEALING. Consider this, a healthy person is going to pay more in premiums than if they got into an accident. Like I wrote in the book, they knock your cost way down if you tell them you do not have insurance. I personally like health sharing programs because they're somewhere in between. I pay $200 per month for my health sharing program. This covers me (they call it sharing) up to $1M in the event of an emergency. I have a course on all this in my virtual membership.

AFTER A SCAN ON MY SPINE, MY DOCTOR SAYS THAT I HAVE STENOSIS. CAN YOU TREAT THIS?

No. We do not treat anything. Treatment is a medical monopoly game. What we do is teach HEAD TO TOE HEALING so that you can get your body back into alignment so it can heal itself. Muscles move bones, therefore you don't have a spine issue, you have a muscle issue. Your muscles have bullied you and have pulled your spine in an odd direction that has created a narrowing which of course creates a slew of new symptoms. Furthermore, you have all sorts of nutritional deficiencies that are making the vertebrae and the cartilage weak. Now, based on my teachings, you have made a mistake. How? You went to the doctor and got tested. The more they test, the more they find. Now, it's stuck in your programming that you have a dis-ease called "stenosis" and that just sounds scary. What was the point? All they did was "zoom in" and look at a part of your spine instead of your muscles, feet, knees, hips, shoulders, neck, nutritional profile, stomach acid, mental health etc. Their solution is now going to be drugs, injections and surgeries, whereas in my membership, I'm teaching you HEAD TO TOE HEALING. It's your choice.

Want to ask me a question?

I'm LIVE every Tuesday at 6pm EST on my main Youtube channel.

www.youtube.com/@CallDrReese

About The Author

Dr. Kevin Reese has helped thousands of people around the world reclaim their health since 2010. He has the most healing results ever captured on video.

While he has a PhD in nutrition and a ton of certifications in other modalities, it's actually his self-study that made him different from everyone else. One day, Dr. Reese had an epiphany that the reason people aren't healing is that schools teach individual parts of the body. After this epiphany, he went on to study the brain, the spine, the pelvis, the gut, the blood, the lymph, the eyes, the feet etc. Learning how it all connected with each other, he made the entire body his specialty and created a new practice called, HEAD TO TOE HEALING. This new approach to health is showcased in his book, PEACE OVER PAIN which has been sold all over the world.

Once he applied HEAD TO TOE HEALING to his clients, the results came pouring in! While most social media influencers are good talkers, Dr. Reese and his team actually captured it all on camera, which verifies that his system works.

His success in healing others is a major reason that he's attacked on and off social media. Dr. Reese has been canceled from social media platforms, shut down at banks, and receives numerous threats from strangers. He is often called a charlatan, a quack, and a grifter.

Through all the controversy and drama, Dr. Reese has become beloved all around the world with half a million followers on social media and dedicated fans who travel long distances to meet him during his annual seminar. Due to all the attacks, he has retired from taking clients and now operates a subscription-based membership that educates people on HEAD TO TOE HEALING.

Learn More → www.DRKEVINREESE.com